T0256170

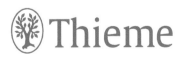

Patient and Family-Centered Speech–Language Pathology and Audiology

Carly Meyer, PhD
Postdoctoral Research Fellow
School of Health and Rehabilitation Sciences
The University of Queensland
Brisbane, Queensland, Australia

Nerina Scarinci, PhD
Associate Professor and Head of Speech Pathology
School of Health and Rehabilitation Sciences
The University of Queensland
Brisbane, Queensland, Australia

Louise Hickson, PhD
Associate Dean External Engagement
Faculty of Health and Behavioural Sciences
The University of Queensland
Brisbane, Queensland, Australia

40 illustrations

Thieme
New York • Stuttgart • Delhi • Rio de Janeiro

Acquisitions Editor: Delia K. DeTurris
Managing Editor: Prakash Naorem
Director, Editorial Services: Mary Jo Casey
Production Editor: Shivika
International Production Director: Andreas Schabert
Editorial Director: Sue Hodgson
International Marketing Director: Fiona Henderson
International Sales Director: Louisa Turrell
Senior Vice President and Chief Operating
   Officer: Sarah Vanderbilt
President: Brian D. Scanlan

Library of Congress Cataloging-in-Publication Data is
available from the publisher

© 2019 Thieme Medical Publishers, Inc.

Thieme Publishers New York
333 Seventh Avenue, New York, NY 10001 USA
+1 800 782 3488, customerservice@thieme.com

Thieme Publishers Stuttgart
Rüdigerstrasse 14, 70469 Stuttgart, Germany
+49 [0]711 8931 421, customerservice@thieme.de

Thieme Publishers Delhi
A-12, Second Floor, Sector-2, Noida-201301
Uttar Pradesh, India
+91 120 45 566 00, customerservice@thieme.in

Thieme Publishers Rio de Janeiro
Thieme Publicações Ltda.
Edifício Rodolpho de Paoli, 25° andar
Av. Nilo Peçanha, 50 – Sala 2508
Rio de Janeiro 20020-906 Brasil
+55 21 3172-2297

Cover design: Thieme Publishing Group
Typesetting by Thomson Digital, India

Printed in USA by King Printing Company, Inc.   5 4 3 2 1

ISBN 978-1-62623-503-8

Also available as an e-book:
eISBN 978-1-62623-920-3

Important note: Medicine is an ever-changing science undergoing continual development. Research and clinical experience are continually expanding our knowledge, in particular our knowledge of proper treatment and drug therapy. Insofar as this book mentions any dosage or application, readers may rest assured that the authors, editors, and publishers have made every effort to ensure that such references are in accordance with **the state of knowledge at the time of production of the book.**

Nevertheless, this does not involve, imply, or express any guarantee or responsibility on the part of the publishers in respect to any dosage instructions and forms of applications stated in the book. **Every user is requested to examine carefully** the manufacturers' leaflets accompanying each drug and to check, if necessary in consultation with a physician or specialist, whether the dosage schedules mentioned therein or the contraindications stated by the manufacturers differ from the statements made in the present book. Such examination is particularly important with drugs that are either rarely used or have been newly released on the market. Every dosage schedule or every form of application used is entirely at the user's own risk and responsibility. The authors and publishers request every user to report to the publishers any discrepancies or inaccuracies noticed. If errors in this work are found after publication, errata will be posted at www.thieme.com on the product description page.

Some of the product names, patents, and registered designs referred to in this book are in fact registered trademarks or proprietary names even though specific reference to this fact is not always made in the text. Therefore, the appearance of a name without designation as proprietary is not to be construed as a representation by the publisher that it is in the public domain.

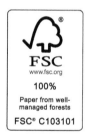

Contents

Contents

3   Getting the Environment Ready for Patient- and Family-Centered Care   46
Nerina Scarinci, Carly Meyer

4   Planning a Patient- and Family-Centered Approach to Service Delivery   70
Carly Meyer, Nerina Scarinci

5   Identifying Patient and Family Member Needs through Assessment   94

Louise Hickson, Tanya Rose, Nerina Scarinci, and Carly Meyer

6   Meeting Patient and Family Member Needs through Collaborative Management Planning   114

Louise Hickson, Carly Meyer, Nerina Scarinci

7   Consideration of Cultural and Linguistic Diversity in Patient- and Family-Centered Care   134

Nerina Scarinci, Carly Meyer, Leanne Sorbello

Videos

Video 1.1: How does your communication disability impact your everyday life?

Video 1.2: How has your communication disability impacted your education or employment?

Video 1.3: Motivation for becoming an audiologist.

Video 1.4: What does patient- and family-centered care mean to you?

Video 1.5: Patient and family member preferences for patient- and family-centered care.

Video 1.6: What positive outcomes have you seen from patient- and family-centered care?

Video 1.7: What does patient- and family-centered care mean for your practice?

Video 2.1: Tips for being a patient- and family-centered clinician.

Video 2.2: Pediatric case history 1.

Video 2.3: Pediatric case history 2.

Video 2.4: Addressing concerns.

Video 2.5: Rapport building.

Video 3.1: Transforming a pediatric clinical environment.

Video 3.2: Transforming an adult clinical environment.

Video 3.3: How can we prepare our clinical rooms for patient- and family-centered care?

Video 3.4: What challenges have you experienced implementing patient- and family-centered care into the clinic?

Video 4.1: How do families benefit from clinician-led parent groups?

Video 5.1: Applying the ICF to your patient- and family-centered assessment.

Video 5.2: What are your tips for setting up and carrying out a patient- and family-centered assessment?

Video 5.3: How can we better understand the lives our patients and families live and what their communication needs are?

Video 5.4: How does your hearing loss form or impact the way you provide care as an audiologist?

Video 6.1: How has your own hearing impairment given you insight into the value of patient-centered care from a client's perspective?

Video 6.2: What advice do you have for working with young children and their families so that our management is patient- and family-centered?

Video 7.1: Defining cultural and linguistic diversity.

Video 7.2: How can clinicians be culturally responsive when working with families from a culturally and linguistically diverse (CALD) background?

Video 7.3: Cultural considerations for patient- and family-centered care (PFCC) across the clinical journey when working with Iranian and Malaysian families.

Video 7.4: Considerations for working with families from a Chilean background.

Video 7.5: How does family-centered practice vary across cultures?

Video 7.6: Advice for working with a family from a culturally and linguistically diverse (CALD) background you are not familiar with.

Foreword

The provision of health care is changing throughout the world. Forces such as technological advancements, generational differences, reimbursement policy, and patient choice are driving what was once a purely medical model of service delivery to a more biopsychosocial approach to care. More and more patients are self-managing their health seeking out mobile applications for diagnosis and treatment, reviewing findings and recommendations online, directly participating with their healthcare providers, and demanding outcome evidence when treatment options are presented.

This trend is not exclusive to health care but is simultaneously occurring in the field of education. Parents are more involved today than ever in the education and services available for their children from infancy through adulthood. Institutions and individual service providers are finding that they must adapt their programs and services to include parental participation in their processes. As with health care, teachers and clinicians must rethink the traditional styles of service provision and develop techniques that can assure positive outcomes.

One unifying group with a significant presence in both the health care and educational arenas is of speech–language pathologists and audiologists. They work tirelessly within an ever-changing system to meet the communication needs of their patients. With the ever-increasing call for treatment evidence, these professionals continue to develop assessment and treatment protocols based on outcomes. What has now become apparent is that patient- and family-centered care is a vital component of improving treatment satisfaction and measurable success.

This is not a future look where health care and education are headed; it is, in fact, the very nature of service provision today. If speech–language pathologists and audiologists are to survive and flourish in these challenging environments, they must embrace the concepts that are already proven to impact the services they provide. It is time to stop thinking patient- and family-centered care is a good idea, rather welcome it into everyday practice. And, improve the experience for patients, families, and clinicians, while achieving the goals and objectives of assessment and treatment.

Drs. Meyer, Scarinci, and Hickson have recognized the importance of the role of patient- and family-centered care in the educational training of speech–language pathologists and audiologists with this new textbook, *Patient and Family-Centered Speech–Language Pathology and Audiology*. They have acknowledged the importance of the subject and realize that it must be incorporated into the educational curriculum for our future professionals. I equate the inclusion of this topic in this educational training with the importance of learning about treatment approaches to communication disorders, goals and objectives, and professional issues and ethics. It is an area that crosses over all aspects of professional training.

The authors have taken a creative approach to presenting the material in this publication by developing it as a handbook that can help guide the student through the process of developing a patient- and family-centered mindset. The book is broken into seven content areas that prepare the student with both scientific evidence of the importance of the subject and practical information for implementation. They have invited an impressive array of international authors to add personal experiences and suggestions to each chapter of the book, giving the student concrete examples of implementation of the concepts expressed in each of the chapters.

The book opens with a chapter dedicated to laying the foundation for the concept of patient- and family-centered care. That is, it provides both underlying principles and scientific research on the topic. The authors carefully show that the patient- and family-centered care is not just a "feel-good" approach to assessment and treatment, rather a proven technique with evidence to back up the concept. With this in mind, the chapters that follow take on a relevant role in providing the student with the information needed to develop the skills necessary for the implementation.

Subsequent chapters such as Chapters 2, 3, and 4 reinforce the ideals presented in Chapter 1 and prepare the student for his/her journey to patient- and family-centeredness. It is here where the reader is introduced to the clinical mindset and the processes necessary to be patient- and family-inclusive. It is important to remember that inviting a family member into the clinical experience alone does not complete the process, and there are many steps necessary prior to that first patient visit. These chapters essentially set the stage for the future patient encounters.

Chapters 5 and 6 are dedicated to the actual patient interaction and the importance of shared decision making, mutual understanding, and management collaboration. It is here where the students are presented with the idea that goal setting should be determined with the input of both the patient and family. It is not just the clinician telling the patient or family member what to do, rather deciding together what the best strategies are for the individual patient and the family unit. Once the goals are determined as a group and an understanding has been reached, each participant will decide what his or her role will be in the process for achieving the objectives. In my view, it is here where the heart and soul of patient- and family-centered care lives, and in this section, the authors provide a comfortable home.

The book concludes with a chapter dedicated to concerns related to cultural and linguistic diversity. As clinicians, we must always be sensitive and responsive to the needs of our patients and their families. In a book related to patient- and family-centered care, the authors are mindful of the specific individual beliefs and behaviors associated with diverse cultures that include perhaps the concept of family itself. As students begin to embrace the idea of patient- and family-centered care, an understanding of the issues regarding cultural and linguistic diversity must be held paramount.

As a clinician, consumer of research, and an academic, I was very pleased to learn about the preparation of this textbook. I have lectured many times on this very topic to practicing speech–language pathologists and audiologists and have believed that it was necessary for patient- and family-centered care to be infused into academic professional education and training as part of student preparation. This book will provide students with the background and knowledge to develop the skills necessary to practice. If I had my way, patient- and family-centered care would be a free-standing required course in all health-related curriculum. However, for the time being, I am thrilled that this textbook will allow it to be offered to speech–language pathology and audiology students. I am honored to have been asked to prepare this foreword in particular, by authors whose work I continue to admire.

Joseph Montano, EdD
Audiologist
Weill Cornell Medical College
New York, New York

Acknowledgments

We are incredibly grateful for all the support we have received from our beautiful families, friends, colleagues, and collaborators throughout the process of producing this book. We could not have achieved this without you! Our book writing journey began with a serendipitous conversation with Thieme at an American Academy of Audiology conference in the United States and further developed with our colleagues in the Communication Disability Centre in the School of Health and Rehabilitation Sciences at The University of Queensland, Australia. After many fruitful discussions, we realized that the best approach for achieving patient- and family-centered care in speech–language pathology and audiology practice would be a practical guide for students. Having recognized that there are many experts in patient- and family-centered care in both clinical practice and research, from the very beginning we were committed to capturing this expertise in the book and so would like to thank all our contributors from Australia and around the world. This book would not be what it is without your contributions! Finally, we would like to specifically thank Caitlin Barr for her significant involvement in the conceptualization of the book and her support throughout the process. We are so grateful that we could begin this journey with you.

Carly Meyer, PhD
Nerina Scarinci, PhD
Louise Hickson, PhD

Contributors

Akmaliza Ali, PhD
Lecturer in Audiology
Rehabilitation Sciences
National University of Malaysia
Bangi, Selangor, Malaysia

David Allen, MAud
Research Higher Degree Student
School of Health and Rehabilitation Sciences
The University of Queensland
Brisbane, Queensland, Australia

Rebecca Armstrong, PhD
Lecturer in Speech Pathology
School of Health and Rehabilitation Sciences
The University of Queensland
Brisbane, Queensland, Australia

Caitlin Barr, PhD
Chief Executive Officer
Better Hearing Australia Victoria
Melbourne, Victoria, Australia

Michelle Bennett, PhD
Lecturer in Speech Pathology
School of Allied Health
Australian Catholic University
Sydney, New South Wales, Australia

Rebecca Bennett, PhD
Postdoctoral Researcher
Ear Science Institute Australia
Perth, Western Australia, Australia

Caitlin Brandenburg, PhD
Advanced Research Development Officer
Gold Coast Hospital and Health Service
Gold Coast, Queensland, Australia

Teresa Ching, PhD
Researcher
National Acoustic Laboratories
Sydney, New South Wales, Australia

Madeleine Colquhoun, BSpPath
Speech–Language Pathologist
BUSHkids
Brisbane, Queensland, Australia

Katie Ekberg, PhD
Postdoctoral Research Fellow
School of Health and Rehabilitation Sciences
The University of Queensland
Brisbane, Queensland, Australia

Kris English, PhD
Associate Professor in Audiology
The University of Akron/NOAC
Akron, Ohio

Adrian Fuente, PhD
Laboratory Director
Centre de recherche
University of Montreal
Montréal, Québec, Canada

Louise Hickson, PhD
Associate Dean External Engagement
Faculty of Health and Behavioral Sciences
The University of Queensland
Brisbane, Queensland, Australia

Anne Hill, PhD
Senior Lecturer in Speech Pathology
School of Health and Rehabilitation Sciences
The University of Queensland
Brisbane, Queensland, Australia

Annie Hill, PhD
Research Fellow
School of Health and Rehabilitation Sciences
The University of Queensland
Brisbane, Queensland, Australia

Lesley Jones, PhD
Educator
University of Bristol
Bristol, UK

Ian Kneebone, PhD
Professor in Psychology
Graduate School of Health
University of Technology Sydney
Sydney, New South Wales, Australia

Ariane Laplante-Lévesque, PhD
Scientific Communication Specialist
Oticon Medical
Smørum, Denmark

Tara Lewis, BSpPath
Speech–Language Pathologist
Institute for Urban Indigenous Health
Brisbane, Queensland, Australia

Jacki Liddle, PhD
Research Fellow in Occupational Therapy
School of Health and Rehabilitation Sciences
The University of Queensland
Brisbane, Queensland, Australia

Brena Lim, MSc
Speech–Language Pathologist
Singapore Health Services
Third Hospital Ave, Bowyer Block, Singapore

Christopher Lind, PhD
Associate Professor in Audiology
College of Nursing and Health Sciences
Flinders University
Adelaide, South Australia, Australia

Carly Meyer, PhD
Postdoctoral Research Fellow
School of Health and Rehabilitation Sciences
The University of Queensland
Brisbane, Queensland, Australia

Joseph Montano, EdD
Audiologist
Weill Cornell Medical College
New York, New York

Alison Moorcroft, BSpchPath (Hons)
Research Higher Degree Student
School of Health and Rehabilitation Sciences
The University of Queensland
Brisbane, Queensland, Australia

Mansoureh Nickbakht, MSc
Research Higher Degree Student
School of Health and Rehabilitation Sciences
The University of Queensland
Brisbane, Queensland, Australia

Jacqueline Nightingale, BOccThy
Occupational Therapist
Queensland Health
Brisbane, Queensland, Australia

Rebecca Nund, PhD
Lecturer in Speech Pathology
School of Health and Rehabilitation Sciences
The University of Queensland
Brisbane, Queensland, Australia

Rachelle Pitt, PhD
Director of Research and Innovation
West Moreton Health
Queensland Health
Brisbane, Queensland, Australia

Jill Preminger, PhD
Program Director for Audiology
University of Louisville
Louisville, Kentucky

Helen Pryce, PhD
Senior Lecturer in Audiology
Life and Health Sciences
Aston University
Birmingham, UK

Teresa Quinlan, BSc (OT)
Clinic Manager/Educator in Occupational Therapy
School of Health and Rehabilitation Sciences
The University of Queensland
Brisbane, Queensland, Australia

Gordy Rogers, MS
Speech–Language Pathologist
Brooklyn Speech Solutions
New York, New York

Tanya Rose, PhD
Lecturer in Speech Pathology
School of Health and Rehabilitation Sciences
The University of Queensland
Brisbane, Queensland, Australia

Brooke Ryan, PhD
Postdoctoral Research Fellow
School of Health and Rehabilitation Sciences
The University of Queensland
Brisbane, Queensland, Australia

Nerina Scarinci, PhD
Associate Professor and Head of Speech Pathology
School of Health and Rehabilitation Sciences
The University of Queensland
Brisbane, Queensland, Australia

Kirstine Shrubsole, PhD
Lecturer in Speech Pathology
School of Health and Human Sciences
Southern Cross University
Gold Coast, Queensland, Australia

Gurjit Singh, PhD
Senior Research Audiologist and Program Manager
Audiologic and Psychological Research
Sonova
Toronto, Ontario, Canada

Cindy Smith, BAppSc
Hanen Instructor and Australasian Representative
The Hanen Centre
Australia

Leanne Sorbello, BSpThy
Speech–Language Pathologist
"Sounds Fun" Speech Pathology
Brisbane, Queensland, Australia

Barbra Timmer, PhD
Adjunct Senior Research Fellow
School of Health and Rehabilitation Sciences
The University of Queensland
Brisbane, Queensland, Australia

Dani Tomlin, PhD
Audiologist and Clinical Manager
Department of Audiology and Speech Pathology
The University of Melbourne
Melbourne, Victoria, Australia

Bettina Turnbull, MAud
Director of Audiology and Education
Sonova, Asia Pacific
Sydney, New South Wales, Australia

Sarah Verdon, PhD
Senior Lecturer in Speech Pathology
School of Community Health
Charles Sturt University
Albury/Wodonga
New South Wales, Australia

Monique Waite, PhD
Postdoctoral Research Fellow
School of Health and Rehabilitation Sciences
The University of Queensland
Brisbane, Queensland, Australia

Kylie Webb, BSpPath
Speech–Language Pathologist
School of Health and Rehabilitation Sciences
The University of Queensland
Brisbane, Queensland, Australia

Gerard William, MAud
Research Higher Degree Student
Department of Audiology and Speech Pathology
The University of Melbourne
Melbourne, Victoria, Australia

Linda Worrall, PhD
Professor in Speech Pathology
School of Health and Rehabilitation Sciences
The University of Queensland
Brisbane, Queensland, Australia

Jenny Ziviani, PhD
Professor in Occupational Therapy
School of Health and Rehabilitation Sciences
The University of Queensland
Brisbane, Queensland, Australia

Chapter 1

Principles and Outcomes of Patient- and Family-Centered Care

1 Principles and Outcomes of Patient- and Family-Centered Care

Carly Meyer, Nerina Scarinci, Caitlin Barr

Abstract

Speech–language pathology and audiology services are provided in a variety of settings, including health and medical facilities, schools, aged care facilities, private practices, and the community. One commonality, however, across each of these settings is the importance of implementing patient- and family-centered care, and consideration of the wide-ranging impacts of communication disability. This chapter discusses the impacts of communication disability in the context of the World Health Organization's International Classification of Functioning, Disability and Health (ICF) and describes the principles and outcomes of patient- and family-centered care. A new model of patient- and family-centered care that is relevant to speech–language pathology and audiology practice is introduced, with the core principles being (1) an effective therapeutic relationship between the patient, family, and clinician; (2) patient- and family-driven care; and (3) consideration of patient and family biopsychosocial needs, preferences, and context. The documented benefits of patient- and family-centered care for individual patients, family members, clinicians, and health services are explored. The purpose of this chapter is to introduce you to theoretical concepts that will be applied in later chapters.

Keywords: patient-centered care, family-centered care, communication disability, ICF, evidence-based practice

Learning Objectives

In this chapter, student speech–language pathologists and audiologists will learn the following:

1. The broad ranging impacts of communication disability on the lives of patients and families.
2. How the World Health Organization's ICF framework can help to identify the impacts of communication disability on patients and families.
3. The principles of patient- and family-centered care in general health care.
4. The key components of patient- and family-centered care in speech–language pathology and audiology.
5. The evidence for patient- and family-centered care in general health care and speech–language pathology and audiology.

1.1 Introduction to Principles and Outcomes of Patient- and Family-Centered Care

In this chapter, we will set the scene for why it is important that speech–language pathologists and audiologists consistently practice patient- and family-centered care. You will be introduced to the wide range of functional impacts that can result from a communication disability in the context of the World Health Organization's ICF framework.[1] You will then be introduced to the principles and outcomes of patient- and family-centered care, where there will be a discussion of similarities, differences, and points of controversy. Speech–language pathology and audiology services are provided in a variety of settings, including health and medical facilities, schools, aged care facilities, private practices, and the community. While the recipients of speech–language pathology and audiology services are referred to as patients, clients, or consumers, depending on the setting; for the purposes of this book, we will refer to all recipients of services as "patients" irrespective of whether or not they are seen in a health, educational, or private setting. Throughout this book we have embedded a number of student activities and reflective exercises. As you grow and develop as a patient- and family-centered speech–language pathologist or audiologist, you will need to reflect on your practice from time to time, and one way to do this is by starting a journal.

The first step we would like you to take in becoming a patient- and family-centered clinician is to develop a *patient- and family-centered reflective journal.* This journal could take the form of a written notebook, electronic diary, blog, twitter feed, video or audio journal; the list is endless. We would like you to use this journal in your own way; however, you are encouraged to actively use it to record your responses to any student activities or reflective exercises. You may also wish to use this journal to note down any "lightbulb" moments, key resources, or take-home messages that you learn as you work through this book.

1.2 The Functional Impact of Communication Disability

In this book, we are going to follow the journey of three people with communication disability and their family members. Before we introduce you to these three people, we want you to hear, firsthand, how communication disability impacts the everyday lives of patients and their family members. Take a moment to watch this video (**Video 1.1**) to understand the far-reaching impacts of communication disability. Then take a look at ▶ Fig. 1.1, which summarizes these impacts in a visual form through the creation of a word cloud based on

direct quotes from these same patients and family members.

Now, meet Emily, a 23-year-old singer in a local Indie band. She has been singing her entire life. In recent years, she has been performing most Friday and Saturday nights at the local live music venue. She does this mostly because she loves it, and also to support her through her University Music Program. A couple of years ago Emily was diagnosed with vocal nodules and saw a speech–language pathologist in order to learn better vocal hygiene behaviors. Recently, she also started to notice a change in her ability to hear in background noise, and, with the encouragement of her boyfriend Hugh, she had a hearing assessment with an audiologist. The audiologist diagnosed Emily with a mild high-frequency hearing loss consistent with noise exposure. Together, Emily's voice disorder and hearing loss means that Emily is struggling to perform at her regular gigs and it's also affecting her University studies.

Also meet Shane. Shane is a 67-year-old retired teacher. Fifteen years ago, Shane was diagnosed with Parkinson's disease. After receiving the diagnosis, he was left with no choice but to retire early, despite loving his job. He currently lives at home with his wife Lorna, who is 65 years old. Shane and Lorna have three children and seven grandchildren. Most of their family members live nearby; however, they do have one son who lives overseas with his wife and two children. Up until a couple of years ago, Shane was still able to drive himself to his regular weekly Bridge Club, where he enjoyed a counter lunch and a beer or two with his old teaching colleagues. More recently, however, his tremor, and slow shuffling gait have

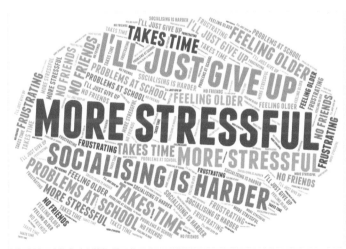

Fig. 1.1 Word cloud of impact of communication disability.

worsened and now he is unable to go out as often as he would like. He has also lost his driver's license because of his deteriorating cognition and thus is no longer able to drive. His diet has recently been modified, and therefore he is no longer able to go out for meals. He is becoming increasingly dependent on his wife, who is finding it difficult to manage the extra responsibilities and stress associated with caring for her husband. As a result of her caring responsibilities, she has also had to stop attending her regular activities with friends as she does not feel that she can leave him at home alone. In addition, Lorna has recently noticed that her hearing has started to deteriorate as she often has difficulty hearing her family and friends around the house, and she is finding it increasingly difficult to hear her husband as his voice remains very soft. She is yet to seek help from an audiologist for her hearing difficulties, not because she hasn't acknowledged her hearing difficulties, rather, she hasn't been able to prioritize it because of her caring responsibilities. Old friends have stopped visiting because they can no longer understand Shane's stories and find that it is becoming increasingly difficult to communicate with Lorna due to her hearing difficulties.

Lastly, it's time to hear Miranda's story. Miranda's son Andrew was diagnosed with autism spectrum disorder (ASD) when he was 3 years of age, after Miranda had long suspected that something wasn't quite right. Andrew was Miranda and Flynn's firstborn child and with no family history of speech or language difficulties, the diagnosis was unexpected. Miranda had a normal pregnancy, and as she lives 2.5 hours from her nearest major hospital, her pregnancy was managed by her local community midwife. Before having Andrew, Miranda was the nurse-in-charge at the local aged care facility, and she returned to work in a part-time capacity after Andrew had his first birthday. After receiving the diagnosis, Miranda

and Flynn decided together that it would be best for their family for her to stop work for a while so they could focus on Andrew's early intervention program. Andrew is now 5 years of age, and communicates using a combination of key word sign and spoken language. Next year, he will be transitioning to school, and Miranda is considering returning to work part-time.

These three case studies represent only a snippet of the patients and family members who speech–language pathologists and audiologists work with on a daily basis. Now, take a moment to view a video (**Video 1.2**) where even more people have shared their stories about the impact of communication disability on their education and employment.

These case studies and videos have demonstrated the wide-ranging impacts that communication disability can have on an individual and their family members. In order to contextualize such impacts, the World Health Organization's ICF framework[1] can be used to provide a holistic, biopsychosocial framework that can help guide your consideration of these impacts.

1.3 The International Classification of Functioning, Disability, and Health

The ICF is a well-known framework, which is used by health professionals worldwide to guide our holistic management of individuals with a communication disability and their family members (▶ Fig. 1.2). The ICF differs from the traditional, biomedical model of health care, where the focus is on the diagnosis and treatment of the disease, so the ICF is often used by speech–language pathologists and audiologists to guide their practice.

The ICF considers the impact of a health condition in two ways. Firstly, it considers the impairments to

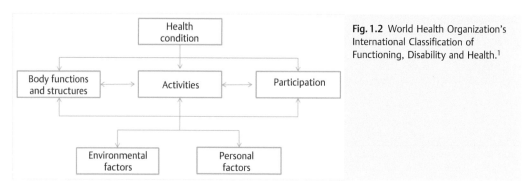

Fig. 1.2 World Health Organization's International Classification of Functioning, Disability and Health.[1]

body functions and structures. Body functions are the physiological functions of the body systems, and body structures are the anatomical parts of the body; impairments are present when there is a problem, deviation, or loss in the body function or structure.[1] The ICF also considers an individual's ability to execute a task or action in an *activity*, and *participate* in a life situation. The negative impacts of a health condition can result in activity limitations and participation restrictions whereby individuals experience difficulties executing activities and involving themselves in life situations.[1] Secondly, the ICF takes into account the social aspects of disability by acknowledging contextual factors such as the impact of the *environment* on a person's functioning, and *personal factors* that enable or disable a person with a health condition.[1] Environmental factors can include factors in the individual's most immediate environment (e.g., products and technology, support and relationships), as well as factors in the general environment (e.g., services, systems, and policies). Personal factors, although not classified in the ICF, consist of factors which incorporate the particular background of an individual's life, such as gender, race, age, coping styles, and educational background.[1]

> ### Helpful Tip
>
> The ICF can be used as a framework for conceptualizing a patient's functioning and for classifying and *coding* impairments, activity limitations, participation restrictions, and environmental barriers and facilitators. The World Health Organization has an online version of the ICF which can be used to explore the breadth of codes which may be relevant for any given patient and his or her family member. Take a look at what this resource can offer you in ensuring you address the entire biopsychosocial functioning of those you care for:
> http://apps.who.int/classifications/icfbrowser/

The clinician's influence over factors in the Environment is often underestimated, and as such, will be the focus of Chapters 2 and 3. For example, the health professional's own skills and individual attitudes, as well as the physical design and setup of the clinical environment, and the products and technology available for both communication and education, can shape how the person with the communication disability experiences the disability. Other environmental factors include all individuals with whom the person with communication disability has a significant relationship, including immediate family, extended family, friends, and acquaintances, and, importantly, the attitudes of these individuals. The ICF also recognizes "third-party disability"—the negative impacts family members and friends experience as a result of the health condition of their significant others—as an environmental factor.[1] Third-party disability acknowledges that family members and friends can experience changes in functioning, including changes to their activities and ability to participate in life situations, because they may be caring for a significant other, making adaptations as a result of their significant other's disability, or because their significant other's disability affects the things they like to do. The concept of third-party disability has been clearly acknowledged in the context of communication disability, specifically, for family members of patients with aphasia,[2] dementia,[3] and hearing impairment.[4]

The best way to fully appreciate the potential application of the ICF to speech–language pathology and audiology is to consider how you would apply the ICF to a patient with a communication disability. ▶ Fig. 1.3 and ▶ Fig. 1.4 illustrate the application of the ICF to Shane and his wife, Lorna, respectively. These figures clearly summarize the background information provided earlier in this chapter about Shane and Lorna. Summarizing the background information in the context of the ICF highlights the wide-ranging impacts of communication disability and the need for holistic intervention.

> ### Student Activity 1.2: Putting the ICF into Practice with Emily and her Family
>
> To increase your familiarity with the ICF framework and appreciate how it can be used to develop a holistic understanding of the impact of communication disability, take a moment to reflect on Emily, the 23-year-old singer and University student you read about earlier in this chapter. Emily has vocal nodules and a mild high-frequency hearing loss. She performs most Friday and Saturday nights at the local live music venue and is completing a music degree at University. Her boyfriend Hugh is very supportive.
>
> Identify how each component of the ICF may be relevant to Emily's functioning and include these in a figure like ▶ Fig. 1.3.

5

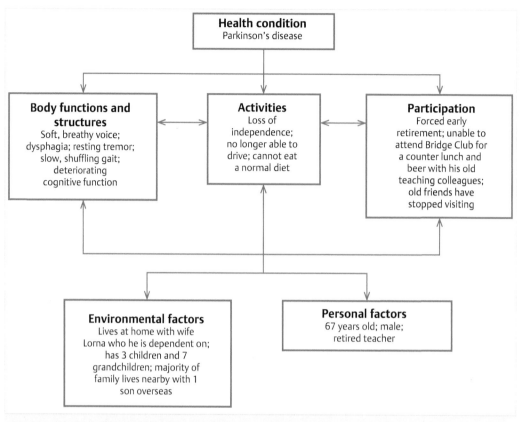

Fig. 1.3 Application of the World Health Organization's International Classification of Functioning, Disability and Health to Shane.

Just like you did with Emily, take a moment to reflect on Miranda, the mother of Andrew who has autism spectrum disorder. How has Andrew's diagnosis impacted Miranda's life?

Identify how each component of the ICF may be relevant to Miranda's third-party functioning and include these in a figure like ▶ Fig. 1.4.

Hopefully these activities have highlighted the importance of applying a biopsychosocial approach to the management of patients with a communication disability and their family. Interestingly though, despite the benefits of taking a biopsychosocial approach, to date, the ICF framework has not necessarily been applied consistently in real-world speech–language pathology and audiology. Joseph Montano describes his perspective on how speech–language pathologists and audiologists are transitioning from a medical model to a biopsychosocial model of service delivery. (See box on "A Word from a Clinical Expert: Establishing a Biopsychosocial Model of Service Delivery").

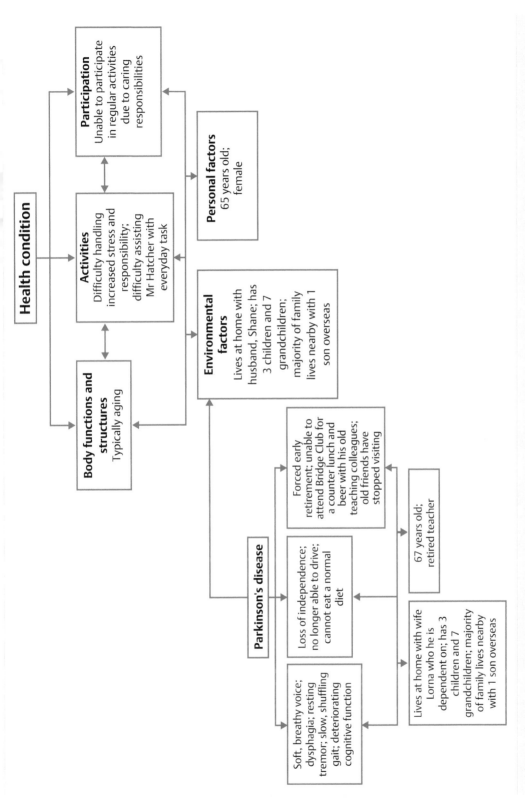

Fig. 1.4 Application of the World Health Organization's International Classification of Functioning, Disability and Health to Shane's wife, Lorna and her experience of third-party disability.

Joseph Montano, Audiologist, United States

All too often, the practice of audiology and speech–language pathology follows what has been termed a medical model of service delivery. That is, the practice becomes curative in nature. A patient with a communication disability presents himself or herself to a speech–language pathologist or audiologist who attempts to solve the problem. Recommendations are based on the formal, standardized assessment, and in order to resolve the communication disability, an impairment-focused intervention is recommended. Essentially, the patient is removed from the equation and the results from the formal, standardized assessment become the primary basis for the recommended treatment. The medical model is a top-down approach, where the clinician is seen as the expert of the patient's communication disability. The medical approach, while necessary and effective in the treatment of acute health crises, is not effective when dealing with a biopsychosocial condition such as communication disability. Clinicians continue to practice in this manner with many of them even wearing white laboratory coats for consultations.

Delivering a biopsychosocial practice requires the establishment of a partnership between the clinician, patient, and the patient's family. The patient and his or her family are the experts of the communication disability. Together, problems associated with communication difficulties can be identified and goals for treatment can be determined. This model of service delivery is rehabilitative in nature and recommended for individuals with chronic health conditions, which is often the case for communication disability. By reframing the patient and family experience, the clinician can build successful relationships, establish trust, and pursue rehabilitative objectives.

The need to take a biopsychosocial approach to addressing the impacts of communication disability requires a certain type of health professional who has the patient's best interests at heart. For some of you, this might have been the key reason why you entered speech–language pathology or audiology. For others, this might be part of your journey to becoming an effective health professional. Now it's time to hear directly from an audiology student in Australia about why she decided to become a health professional.

I think it's fair to say that most of us don't know what we'd like to do for the rest of our lives. I think that a lot of us believe that we need to know what we did like to do as soon as we leave high school but the reality of it is that most of us don't know exactly what we want. I knew that I wanted to be a health professional but I didn't know specifically what I wanted to do. I started my university journey in science. Being such a diverse degree, I thought science would give me a solid foundation, challenge me, and also give me some time to think about what I wanted to do… and if I didn't know then there was always the exciting prospect of doing research! I originally thought that I would go into medicine because that seemed like the most obvious choice; however, I knew that wasn't my passion. Towards the end of my science degree I was searching for something else that I could see myself doing.

Two things led me towards audiology. First of all, I tagged along to an information night for prospective audiology students with a friend of mine. Audiology is a small profession, so it's not unusual that people know very little about it. I was intrigued by the amount of change audiologists could make to someone's life. Hearing is never really at the forefront of health care. In fact, most people think the loss of hearing is an inevitable process of aging and we just have to deal with it as it comes. Few people look at hearing loss as a serious condition, but hearing loss can be an extremely debilitating condition. It can completely isolate people as they withdraw from social activities and can feel alone in their journey. Hearing loss can build frustrations and greatly strain relationships. Audiological rehabilitation can make significant changes to someone's quality of life and it isn't just about hearing aids.

My second path to audiology was much more personal. A relative of mine had her first baby and he came into the world without the ability to hear his mother's voice. He was born profoundly deaf and to a couple who had never had a child before; you can imagine it was a lot to take on board. When he turned 3, his parents made the decision to go ahead with a cochlear implant…and what an amazing experience it was to sit in that room with them and see his whole world come to life. There are just some experiences that you can't explain in words. As cliché as it sounds, that was the moment I knew that I made the right decision to be an audiologist.

To hear why another student, who actually has a hearing loss himself, chose a career in audiology, take a look at **Video 1.3**.

The reason why it is important to reflect on what it takes to be an effective health professional is because that is what should drive us all to be the best clinician that we can. We acknowledge, however, that everyone's story is different—we're sure there are others who have entered the profession with similar motivations to Stephanie, as well as other reasons. Now is a great opportunity for you to reflect on why you decided to become a health professional.

Irrespective of individual differences in the motivations people have for becoming a health professional, to fulfil our professional obligations and meet the diverse needs of patients and family, it is important that we align these motivations with the principles of patient- and family-centered care.

1.4 Principles of Patient- and Family-Centered Care

Patient-centered care has its roots in psychological counseling, where Carl Rogers acknowledged the central role of the therapeutic relationship with patients.[5] He saw the relationship between patient and practitioner as inseparable from the clinical encounter. Since the 1960s, the notion of patient-centered care has extended to mainstream medicine and health care, and has transformed into a conceptual framework that promotes high quality, holistic care where the patient is seen as, and encouraged to be, an active participant in his or her own health care.[6] Unsurprisingly, this transformation has seen many attempts at defining, understanding, framing, measuring, and implementing patient-centered care.

One such transformation relates to the different terms used to describe patient-centered care. Carl Rogers originally coined the term "client-centered care," which aligned with the typical terminology used in psychological therapy. The term "patient-centered care" gained popularity in the 1980s to the 2000s due to the increase in its application to medicine and nursing and is the term that has been used throughout this book. Patient-centered care is described by the Institute of Medicine as an approach to patient care that is respectful and responsive to the needs and individual values of any and all patients.[7]

The principles of patient-centered care were recently explored in a systematic review and concept analysis of definitions of patient-centered care,[8] and later verified in a review by the same research team.[9] Scholl et al[8] and Zill et al[9] described patient-centeredness as a concept containing four principles, six activities, and five enablers. The four principles identified in the review provide the foundation for delivering patient-centered care, with the first principle focusing on essential characteristics needed by a clinician in order to successfully implement patient-centered care, that is, being respectful, empathetic, honest, committed to the patient, and self-reflective. Secondly, patient-centered care places emphasis on the importance of the clinician–patient relationship that reflects trust, connection, mutual caring, mutual knowledge, and mutual understanding of roles and responsibilities. Thirdly, in patient-centered care, the clinician must understand that the patient is a unique person who has individual needs, preferences, values, beliefs, concerns, ideas, and expectations, which must be considered when exploring the functional impact of the patient's disease experience. Lastly, patient-centered care acknowledges the importance of taking a biopsychosocial perspective of the patient's condition, including an understanding of the patient's illness in the context of his or her unique biological, psychological, and social context,[8] which aligns nicely with the application of the ICF that we introduced earlier.

The activities described by Scholl et al[8] that underpin the principles of patient-centered care are inherently within the control of the individual clinician. The six activities include, bilateral sharing of patient information that is individually tailored; patient involvement through active participation and engagement in decision making; patient empowerment through the promotion of autonomy and self-management; and emotional and physical support through listening and responding to psychosocial concerns. Finally, involvement of family and friends according to patient preferences was identified as a key activity of patient-centered care, whereby family and friends are provided with information, involved in decision making, and provided with support to address their own unique needs.[8]

In implementing patient-centered care, it is also important to acknowledge the factors that enable the occurrence of patient-centered care and these typically occur at the service level. In their systematic review, Scholl et al[8] identified five enablers to patient-centered care, with arguably the most pertinent being clinician–patient communication, incorporating both verbal and nonverbal communication behaviors such as the use of open-ended questions, paraphrasing key information, adequate eye contact, and acknowledging the patient story through nodding. Other enablers include integration of medical and nonmedical care, coordination and continuity of care, team work and team building, and access to care,[8] although the final two enablers were later found to be less pertinent through the review process.[9]

While "patient-centered care" represents a significant shift away from the medical model, and does acknowledge the importance of involving the family, definitions and descriptions of patient-centered care have not necessarily highlighted the centrality of the patient's family and their biopsychosocial context in this process. For this reason, we turn to the pediatric literature where the term "family-centered care" is frequently used. Family-centered care represents an extension of

A Word from a Research Expert: How Do Young Adults Define "Family"?

David Allen, Audiologist, Australia

The period of life following adolescence, referred to as "young adulthood" or "emerging adulthood,"[13] is one marked by significant change across a range of domains of life. In Australia, while most young people entering emerging adulthood do so while living with one or more parents, by the age of 25, a large proportion will have moved away to live alone, with friends, or with a spouse or other romantic partner.[14]

The absence of parents, grandparents, or other siblings in the day-to-day life of a young person may lead to these emotional, physical, and economical support relationships being filled by friends, romantic partners, or other people with whom the young person does not have a biological relationship, known as the "logical family"[15] or the "functional family."[16] When working with young people living with communication difficulties or ongoing disabilities, engaging with family is particularly important,[17] as well-informed and engaged family has an important support and facilitation role in the patient's care on an ongoing basis.[18] This role may be particularly important for young people with communication difficulties moving out of home and developing new members of their logical family, as moving away from home may remove parents or siblings from contributing to the ongoing support of communication rehabilitation.

The rapid pace of change in various domains of a young person's life may further complicate the definition of family, as who a young person chooses to bring to an appointment may change over a relatively short period of time. In particular, over the course of emerging adulthood, young people develop romantic competence, a process marked by an increase in the exclusivity, intimacy, and duration of romantic relationships. As this stability emerges, however, relationships may be subject to significant change over relatively short periods of time.[19] As a result, when working with emerging adult patients, the existence or composition of a primary romantic relationship cannot be assumed from appointment to appointment.

This is further complicated by broader social changes in the approaches to and definitions of primary relationships over the last several decades, as fewer young people expect primary romantic relationships to be permanent.[20] Young people are also more aware of, and more accepting of, same-sex families,[21] polyamory,[22] and other nontraditional relationship and family structures.[23] This brings the "self-definition" of family referenced by Kaakinen et al[24] to the fore, as young people explore and develop personal conceptions of family that may be very different from the traditional "nuclear family" that may have been appropriate for their parents or grandparents. As a result, when defining the family for the purposes of delivering care, practitioners should be led by patients, empowering them to clearly articulate who they consider to constitute their family, allowing flexibility as this definition may change over time, and working to incorporate these definitions into their practice without negative judgment.

patient-centered care with the key difference being that in family-centered care, the entire family unit is recognized as the recipient of care. Although family-centered care has traditionally been used exclusively in the pediatric context, it has recently been extended to include adults and their network, emphasizing the importance of the familial (and social) context in which individuals exist.

Epley et al[10] conducted a systematic review of family-centered definitions to provide a consensus definition for family-centered care. Epley and colleagues identified five key elements to family-centered care, including: (1) family as the unit of attention; (2) family choice; (3) family strengths; (4) family–professional relationship; and (5) individualized family services. The first element "family as the unit of attention" highlights the importance of considering *all* family members' needs when planning, delivering, and evaluating services. Of course, we would like to stress that although some people may misconstrue family-centered care as devaluing the patient with the health condition, the true ethos of family-centered care values both the patient with the health condition and his or her family members equally. Family choice encapsulates patient and family choice regarding the definition of family, joint decision making, nature of the relationship between the family and the clinician, confidentiality and sharing of information, and goal setting.[11] Family strengths were highlighted by Epley et al[10] as a key component of family-centered care, with family strengths being identified and incorporated into all aspects of management planning. Similar to patient-centered care, the practice of family-centered care relies on the establishment and maintenance of a true partnership between patients, families, and professionals. Finally, family-centered care acknowledges the importance of individualizing services for patients and their families, based on the unique needs and preferences of the family unit. Importantly, when we refer to "family" within the context of family-centered care, we refer to "two or more individuals who depend on one another for emotional, physical, and economical support" with the members of the family being self-defined.[12]

The broader definition of family may be especially relevant for younger adults who are at a stage of transition from childhood to adulthood, and thus also may be at a stage of transition regarding who they consider their family to be. David Allen from The University of Queensland has conducted research with young adults with hearing loss to explore how patient- and family-centered care applies to this population. (See box on previous page "A Word from a Research Expert: How Do Young Adults Define "Family"?").

1.5 A Model of Patient- and Family-Centered Care in Speech–Language Pathology and Audiology

The above summaries of patient- and family-centered care have identified a number of commonalities between these two models of care. Despite these commonalities, to date, there has not been a single model of care, which brings together the commonalities, and which places equal emphasis on the patient with the health condition and the family. To overcome this gap, we propose an integrated model of patient- and family-centered care where the needs of the entire family unit are considered (▶ Fig. 1.5). This model has three core principles: (1) an effective therapeutic relationship between the patient, family, and clinician; (2) patient- and family-driven care; and (3) consideration of patient and family biopsychosocial needs, preferences, and context. From this point on, patient- and family-centered care will be discussed according to these core principles, and we will use the term patient- and family-centered care (PFCC). The application of these principles to speech–language pathology and audiology practice is discussed in the remainder of this chapter and throughout each chapter of the book.

1.5.1 An Effective Therapeutic Relationship between the Patient, Family, and Clinician

Much like all conceptualizations of PFCC, the quality of the communication and relationship between the patient who seeks health care, his or her family, and the clinician is a high priority in speech–language pathology and audiology. Accordingly, this has been included as the first core principle of PFCC. As a speech–language pathologist or audiologist practicing PFCC, you are responsible for prioritizing the development of a trusting, caring, and respectful relationship with both your patient and his or her family. Central to this therapeutic relationship are strong communication skills, both verbal and nonverbal. In addition, as a patient- and family centered clinician, you must give consideration to the environment in which you conduct your clinical

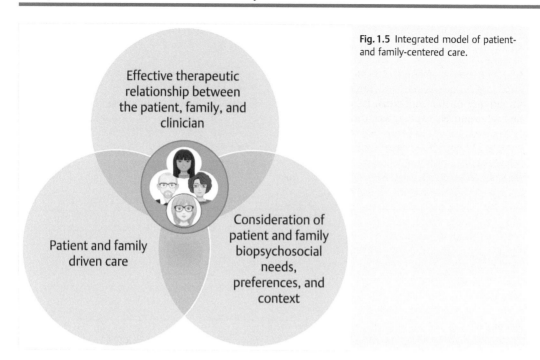

Fig. 1.5 Integrated model of patient- and family-centered care.

Effective therapeutic relationship between the patient, family, and clinician

Consideration of patient and family biopsychosocial needs, preferences, and context

Patient and family driven care

services. These concepts are explored further in Chapters 2 and 3, where communication skills and the importance of preparing the physical, social, and attitudinal environment to optimize PFCC are discussed.

1.5.2 Patient- and Family-Driven Care

The second core principle of PFCC highlights the importance of balancing the control equally between the patient, family, and clinician and encouraging patients and their families to play an active role in driving their own care. Facilitating patient- and family driven care means that the clinician actively strives towards patient and family empowerment and away from clinician-led decision making and planning. Tools to facilitate patient- and family driven care are discussed in detail in Chapters 4, 5, and 6.

1.5.3 Consideration of Patient and Family Biopsychosocial Needs, Preferences, and Context

To provide PFCC, a clinician should have an in-depth understanding of the patient and family and then ensure that these factors are incorporated into the care provided. Accordingly, the third core principle of PFCC is consideration of the patient's and family's biopsychosocial needs, preferences and context. Patient and family biopsychosocial needs includes an understanding of the holistic impact of the communication disability, as conceptualized by the ICF. Patient and family preferences refer to understanding how a patient and family have worked together in the past, and how they would like to work together in the current context (i.e., how to work towards the goals). Lastly, context refers to having an understanding of the personal and environmental factors influencing how the patient and their family functions (i.e., what are the strengths, barriers and considerations that will impact the success of the service). A specific contextual factor which should be considered in the implementation of any PFCC service is cultural and linguistic diversity. In recognition of the importance of this contextual factor, Chapter 7 is dedicated entirely to being a culturally and linguistically responsive patient- and family-centered clinician. Now that we have described the importance of considering the patient and family's biopsychosocial needs, preferences, and context, let's hear firsthand from Kylie Webb, a speech–language pathologist in Australia, about why the biopsychosocial context is so important when working with children in a patient- and family-centered way (**Video 1.4**).

1.6 General Health Care Evidence for Patient- and Family-Centered Care

Like any model of health care, before implementing PFCC as a speech–language pathologist or audiologist, you must be cognizant of the evidence behind this approach. Evidence-based practice (EBP) is a fundamental tenet of modern day health care and involves the integration of the best available research evidence with the clinician's expertise and the patient's and family's needs, preferences, and context. Below we present the best available research evidence for PFCC; however, in order to practice EBP, you must also take into consideration the biopsychosocial needs,

preferences, and context of your patient and his or her family, as well as your own clinical expertise.

In presenting the evidence for PFCC, we will first look more broadly than speech–language pathology and audiology literature, and go to the general health care literature. Evidence for PFCC centers around four primary areas of outcome: (1) patient-level outcomes; (2) family-level outcomes; (3) clinician-level outcomes; and (4) service-level outcomes. We will discuss each of these areas of outcome separately in the following section. ▶ Fig. 1.6 provides a summary of the key outcomes of PFCC within each of the areas. In this summary, it should be noted that condition-specific improvements were the result of condition-specific, patient- and family-centered interventions (e.g., improved hemoglobin levels were the result of patient- and family-centered diabetes management) and cannot not be generalized across all conditions.

1.6.1 Patient-Level Outcomes

The positive impacts of PFCC are well documented and include improvements in body function and structure, as well as activities and participation for a range of health conditions. With respect to body functions and structures, PFCC has been found to result in less severe delirium, reduced cognitive decline, improved child cognitive and motor development, increased infant weight gain, reduced child and adult body mass index, reduced duration of grief disorders, reduced health complications,

Patient-level outcomes	Family-level outcomes
• Improved health status • Better psychosocial health and quality of life • Decreased activity limitations and participation restrictions • Better child behaviour • Improved self-efficacy • Increased knowledge and improved attitudes • Positive behavioural changes • Better treatment adherence	• Reduced anxiety and depression • Improved coping skills • Increased quality of life and psychosocial well-being • Enhanced knowledge, skills, attitudes, and confidence towards health • Improved caregiving practices • Lower caregiver burden
Clinician-level outcomes	**Service-level outcomes**
• Improved knowledge of patient/family management plan • Improved communication skills • Increased engagement • Greater job satisfaction • Reduced burnout	• Improved communication • Improved continuity of care • Better consumer satisfaction and • experience ratings • Improved efficiency • Reduced healthcare costs • Decreased adverse events • Higher employee retention rates • Fewer malpractice claims • Increased market share

Fig. 1.6 Summary of the benefits of patient- and family-centered care.

improved hemoglobin levels, and improved mental health, including reduced stress and anxiety.[25–46] Improvements in activities and participation include improved walking performance and improved communication skills.[26,42,47,48]

In addition to improved health status, PFCC can result in better outcomes for the patient's psychosocial functioning, including improved quality of life and enhanced social interactions.[27,36,41,46,49–51] There is also documented evidence demonstrating that PFCC results in improvements to children's academic and behavioral skills,[42,52,53] self-efficacy,[54] and knowledge of health conditions and attitudes toward health care interventions in adults.[36,45,54,55] Presumably as a result of improved knowledge and attitudes toward health, PFCC can also promote positive behavior changes in the patient with the health condition, such as, better exercise tolerance,[41] increased physical activity, reduced screen time, improved dietary

behavior,[38,56–59] better diabetes management,[54] as well as improved children's behavior.[39,43,60,61,62] Finally, PFCC has been associated with better adherence to treatment plans[25,46,58] and medications.[58]

1.6.2 Family-Level Outcomes

Consistent with the underlying principle of PFCC to address the needs of the entire family unit, there is a mounting body of evidence in support of positive family-level outcomes, such as reduced parental and family member anxiety and depression,[26,29,39,43,61,63–67] improved coping skills,[65,68] as well as enhanced quality of life and psychosocial well-being.[53,69] Family members have also reported better knowledge, confidence, skills and attitudes toward health conditions and health interventions,[34,53] improved communication,[42,68,70] family relationships,[29,49,60,68,70,71] and family functioning.[66,67,70]

Subsequent to direct impacts on the health and well-being of family members, PFCC also promotes the family members' capacity to provide care for the person with the health condition, e.g., by increasing family members' preparedness and confidence for caregiving,[26,72] especially after discharge;[73] improving their willingness to provide care;[27] empowering families to support the person with the health condition;[74] helping family members to reactivate their role within the family unit;[74] and importantly, reducing caregiver burden.[61,69,75] Specific to parents of children with health conditions, PFCC results in changes to parenting behaviors, such as reduced dysfunctional parenting practices,[52,53,61,62] and improved parenting confidence.[42,62]

1.6.3 Clinician-Level Outcomes

Of growing interest in the literature is the impact of PFCC on clinician outcomes. Importantly, acknowledgement of these outcomes is important in motivating clinicians to implement and continue to practice as a patient- and family-centered clinician. Less research has explicitly explored clinician-level outcomes, but there is evidence that clinicians have a positive attitude toward new PFCC interventions,[55,76] and that patient- and family-centered clinicians have a better understanding of the patient and family's overall management plan,[77] and improve their communication style with patients and family members.[77] Ultimately, evidence suggests that clinicians who are more patient- and family-centered report greater satisfaction and engagement with the caring process[48,78] and reduced professional burnout.[79]

1.6.4 Service-Level Outcomes

An important reason why organizations should adopt a PFCC approach is because it not only results in improved outcomes for the person with the health condition, his or her family, and the clinicians involved in their care, but also, there is clear evidence that it results in improved service-level outcomes. A PFCC approach to health care, by its very nature, has resulted in greater patient and family member involvement in health care,[28,52] and subsequently, improved communication between patients, family members, and clinicians, better matching of care to family preferences and needs, and the development of a therapeutic relationship between all members.[48,68,71,74,80,81] Furthermore, there is evidence in support of a PFCC approach leading to improved clinical processes

and coordination of care,[45,48,55,70,74,75,80] greater patient and family member satisfaction with health services,[45,48,53,59,62,70,76,78,82] and improved confidence in the health care team.[63] Lastly, the implementation of PFCC results in improved access to health care[70,75] and improved efficiency of health services (e.g., reduced readmission rates to hospital, fewer emergency department presentations, and shorter length of stay), resulting in reduced health care costs,[29,44,70,72,73,75,76,78,83–85] decreased adverse events, higher employee retention rates, fewer malpractice claims, and, increased market share.[86]

Keen to Hear More about the Benefits of PFCC?

Refer to CanChild's fact sheet on how family-centered services make a difference, available: https://www.canchild.ca/system/tenon/assets/attachments/000/001/267/original/FCS3.pdf

Student Activity 1.5: Reflections on the Implications of Patient- and Family-Centered Care for Speech–Language Pathology and Audiology Practice

Now that you understand what PFCC is at a conceptual level, and what the outcomes of PFCC are, think back to you and your profession.
1. Write a short reflection (300 words) on what you think the implications for providing, or not providing PFCC are for your profession and society at large.
2. Write a short reflection (300 words) on what you think you are going to find most challenging about being a patient- and family-centered clinician, and what information or support you need to get there.

1.7 Evidence from Speech–Language Pathology and Audiology for Patient- and Family-Centered Care

Now that we have reviewed the general health care evidence for PFCC, let's turn our heads to the world of speech–language pathology and audiology where there is increasing evidence as to the positive outcomes of PFCC. For example, there is evidence that PFCC results in improved patient and family satisfaction with speech–language pathology and audiology services.[87–91] Importantly, not only do patients and families express satisfaction with PFCC, but a growing body of research also indicates that patients and family members also have a strong preference for PFCC. So, let's hear from Gurjit Singh, a Canadian audiologist, about a study he has conducted which explored patient and family member preferences for PFCC (**Video 1.5**). Let's also hear from Kylie Webb again about the positive outcomes she has observed from practicing PFCC with young children and their families (**Video 1.6**).

1.7.1 Patient-Level Outcomes

Research in speech–language pathology and audiology has reported that as a result of PFCC

services, patients feel more engaged with services[92,93] and experience increased self-efficacy, autonomy, and empowerment.[93] At the impairment level, PFCC improves patient communication skills, including speech,[91,94,95] fluency,[96] and receptive and expressive language skills.[91,94,95,97–103] Studies have also reported improvements to patient activities and participation, including conversation skills and use of effective communication strategies,[102,104–106] social communication skills,[95,98,107] early cognitive development and play skills,[98] and academic skills.[95] Importantly, research has shown that, as a result of PFCC, patients with communication disabilities have more success with the generalization and maintenance of communication skills.[108]

The benefits of PFCC in speech–language pathology and audiology also extend to patients' psychosocial functioning, including acceptance of their

---

A Word from a Research Expert: Working toward a Patient- and Family-Centered Research Agenda within a Health Facility

Jenny Ziviani, Occupational Therapist, Australia

There will be work situations in which you may find the rhetoric in strategic planning documents difficult to map against organizational policies, procedures, and practices. It is now well appreciated that involving consumers, individually and at the community level, in health service practices and research improves the outcomes for patients, families, and organizations alike.[112]

In the Australian context, there are a number of examples where guidelines exist that provide practical examples of how patient- and family-centered involvement in research can be operationalized. Here I will focus on health and medical research where the involvement of patients and families as participants is critical to research outcomes and the meaningful translation of interventions into practice. It is with this in mind that the *Involving People in Research: Consumer and Community Health Research Network* was established (http://www.involvingpeopleinresearch.org.au). In their "Purple book" publication, McKenzie and Hanley[113] have made resources readily available to assist clinicians in identifying the range of consumers they need to consider for their specific research endeavors (e.g., individuals receiving health care, consumer organizations, taxpayers/citizens who ultimately pay for services). Working through these very practical guidelines enable researchers to involve patients and families from the very start in order to ensure that what is being planned is both feasible and acceptable to participants.

The extent of consumer and community involvement can also vary depending on the nature of the research being undertaken. At its fullest extent, patients and families can lead the research or be seen as equal partners in the undertaking. This "co-production" approach is a way of not only addressing issues, which are important to participants but also ensuring that the findings are more readily disseminated and translated into practice. To be able to feel confident to contribute to research teams, patients and families benefit from specific training in relation to the research process. The Autism Collaborative Research Centre (www.autismcrc.com.au) established a "Research Academy," which provides a structured program whereby individuals with autism and their families can be provided with the skills necessary to enable them to participate in the design and implementation of research projects. Practical worksheets accompany this training and can be readily accessed (http://www.autismcrc.com.au/inclusive-autism-research). While this training attends to the specific needs of those with autism, more generalized training is also available through the *Involving People in Research: Consumer and Community Health Research Network*. This empowering process enhances the contributions patients and families make to the research process, and allows them to provide their insights appropriately.[114]

disability, and improved adjustment, confidence, self-esteem, self-perception of their own identity, child attachment, and quality of life.[93,95,98,102,104, 106,109,110] Patients have also reported feeling less withdrawn and less discouraged as a result of receiving PFCC services.[105] Improvements in psychological functioning, namely reductions in depression, anxiety, and negative effect, have also been reported as a result of patient- and family-centered speech–language pathology and audiology.[93,95,98,102,110]

1.7.2 Family-Level Outcomes

PFCC in speech–language pathology and audiology can also result in positive outcomes for family members. These outcomes include increased family knowledge about communication disability,[102,109,111] improved knowledge and use of communication strategies,[100,102,107,109] and better parent–child interactions.[97,100] Improvements in family psychosocial and psychological functioning have also been reported, including improved self-confidence, self-esteem, self-perceptions[102,103] and reduced depression,[102] parental stress,[103,108] and third-party disability.[110] Importantly, research also suggests that as a result of receiving PFCC services, families also experience improvements in their quality of life.[87,108]

The benefits from PFCC in speech–language pathology and audiology do not stop at patient- and family-level outcomes however. There are additional benefits to clinicians and services that have not yet been extensively documented. With this in mind, we spoke to Bettina Turnbull, an audiologist in Australia who has experience in implementing PFCC at an organizational level (**Video 1.7**).

Lastly, it is important to remember that you, as speech–language pathologists and audiologists, will be encouraged to contribute to the ongoing evidence base for PFCC, be it as research participants, research collaborators, or research investigators. Of course, in the context of PFCC, research would not be complete without the involvement of patients and families in the process. Jenny Ziviani, an occupational therapist in Australia, shares her passion for involving consumers in the research process. (See box on "A Word from a Research Expert: Working toward a Patient- and Family-Centered Research Agenda within a Health Facility").

1.8 Summary

The implementation of patient- and family-centered care is the cornerstone to quality, holistic health care, and is particularly relevant for you as speech–language pathology and audiology professionals, who will focus on assisting patients and families impacted by communication disability. Key elements of PFCC that must be implemented for it to occur are: (1) building an effective therapeutic relationship between the patient, family, and clinician; (2) encouraging care that is patient and family driven (rather than clinician driven); and (3) considering the total picture of patients' and families' lives by understanding their biopsychosocial needs, preferences, and context as described in the ICF. Being a patient- and family-centered clinician offers great benefits to you, your patients, their families, and your employer. Importantly, it will ensure you will have a long and satisfying career ahead! In the chapters that follow we will elaborate on the practical implementation of PFCC in clinical contexts.

1.9 Reflections

Please respond to the following reflection questions in your PFCC journal:

1. What are the three principles of PFCC in the model?
2. Who can benefit from PFCC?
3. Consider a recent clinical encounter in speech–language pathology or audiology. Reflect on whether or not the patients and their families experienced a biopsychosocial approach or if the focus was more biomedical. What were the signs that helped you identify the approach?

References

[1] World Health Organization. ICF, International Classification of Functioning, Disability and Health. Geneva: World Health Organization; 2001

[2] Grawburg M, Howe T, Worrall L, Scarinci N. Third-party disability in family members of people with aphasia: a systematic review. Disabil Rehabil. 2013; 35(16):1324–1341

[3] Byrne K, Orange JB. Conceptualizing communication enhancement in dementia for family caregivers using the WHO- ICF framework. Adv Speech Lang Pathol. 2005; 7(4):187–202

[4] Scarinci N, Worrall L, Hickson L. The ICF and third-party disability: its application to spouses of older people with hearing impairment. Disabil Rehabil. 2009; 31(25):2088–2100

[5] Rogers C. Client-Centered Therapy: Its Current Practice, Implication, and Theory. Boston, MA: Houghton Mifflin; 1965

[6] Mead N, Bower P. Patient-centredness: a conceptual framework and review of the empirical literature. Soc Sci Med. 2000; 51(7):1087–1110

[7] Committee on Quality of Health Care in America. Crossing the quality chasm: A new health system for the 21st century. Washington, DC: Institute of MEdicine;2001

[8] Scholl I, Zill JM, Härter M, Dirmaier J. An integrative model of patient-centeredness—a systematic review and concept analysis. PLoS One. 2014; 9(9):e107828

[9] Zill JM, Scholl I, Härter M, Dirmaier J. Which dimensions of patient-centeredness matter? Results of a web-based expert Delphi survey. PLoS One. 2015; 10(11):e0141978

[10] Epley P, Summers JA, Turnbull A. Characteristics and trends in family-centered conceptualizations. J Fam Soc Work. 2010; 13(3):269–285

[11] Allen RI, Petr CG. Toward developing standards and measurements for family-centered practice in family support programs. In: Singer GHS, Powers LE, Olson AL, eds. Redefining Family Support. Baltimore, MD: Paul H Brookes Publishing; 1996:57–84

[12] Hanson SMH. Family health care nursing: an introduction. In: Hanson SMH, Gedaly-Duff V, Kaakinen JR, eds. Family Health Care Nursing: Theory, Practice and Research. 3rd ed. Philadelphia, PA: F. A. Davis; 2005:1–38

[13] Arnett JJ. Emerging adulthood. A theory of development from the late teens through the twenties. Am Psychol. 2000; 55(5):469–480

[14] Hillman KJ, Marks GN. Becoming an Adult: Leaving Home, Relationships and Home Ownership among Australian Youth. Camberwell, Victoria: The Australian Centre for Educational Research; 2002

[15] Maupin A. Michael Tolliver Lives. London; Doubleday; 2007

[16] Medalie JH, Cole-Kelly K. The clinical importance of defining family. Am Fam Physician. 2002; 65(7):1277–1279

[17] Dillon H. Hearing Aids. 2nd ed. Turramurra, New South Wales: Boomerang Press; 2012

[18] Committee on hospital care and institute for patient- and family centered care. Patient- and family-centered care and the pediatrician's role. Pediatrics. 2012; 129(2):394–404

[19] Meier A, Allen G. Romantic relationships from adolescence to young adulthood: evidence from the national longitudinal study of adolescent health. Sociol Q. 2009; 50(2):308–335

[20] Orrange RM. The emerging mutable self: gender dynamics and creative adaptations in defining work, family, and the future. Soc Forces. 2003; 82(1):1–34

[21] Twenge JM, Sherman RA, Wells BE. Changes in American adults' reported same-sex sexual experiences and attitudes, 1973–2014. Arch Sex Behav. 2016; 45(7):1713–1730

[22] Barker M. This is my partner, and this is my … partner's partner: constructing a polyamorous identity in a monogamous world. J Constr Psych. 2005; 18(1):75–88

[23] Allen KR, Crosbie-Burnett M. Innovative ways and controversial issues in teaching about families: a special collection on family pedagogy. Fam Relat. 1992; 41(1):9

[24] Kaakinen JR, Gedaly-Duff V, Coehlo DP, Harmon SMH. Family health care nursing: Theory, practice and research. Philadelphia: F.A. Davis Company; 2010

[25] Bahramnezhad F, Asgari P, Zolfaghari M, Farokhnezhad Afshar P. Family-centered education and its clinical outcomes in patients undergoing hemodialysis short running. Iran Red Crescent Med J. 2015; 17(6):e20705

[26] Boltz M, Resnick B, Chippendale T, Galvin J. Testing a family-centered intervention to promote functional and cognitive recovery in hospitalized older adults. J Am Geriatr Soc. 2014; 62(12):2398–2407

[27] Chang AK, Park YH, Fritschi C, Kim MJ. A family involvement and patient-tailored health management program in elderly Korean stroke patients' day care centers. Rehabil Nurs. 2015; 40(3):179–187

[28] Dixon LB, Glynn SM, Cohen AN, et al. Outcomes of a brief program, REORDER, to promote consumer recovery and family involvement in care. Psychiatr Serv. 2014; 65(1):116–120

[29] Ettenberger M, Rojas Cárdenas C, Parker M, Odell-Miller H. Family-centred music therapy with preterm infants and their parents in the Neonatal Intensive Care Unit (NICU) in Colombia—a mixed-methods study. Nord J Music Ther. 2016; 25(1):21–22

[30] Falbe J, Cadiz AA, Tantoco NK, Thompson HR, Madsen KA. Active and healthy families: a randomized controlled trial of a culturally tailored obesity intervention for Latino children. Acad Pediatr. 2015; 15(4):386–395

[31] Kissane DW, Zaider TI, Li Y, et al. Randomized controlled trial of family therapy in advanced cancer continued into bereavement. J Clin Oncol. 2016; 34(16):1921–1927

[32] Martínez-Velilla N, Garrués-Irisarri M, Ibañez-Beroiz B, et al. An exercise program with patient's involvement and family support can modify the cognitive and affective trajectory of acutely hospitalized older medical patients: a pilot study. Aging Clin Exp Res. 2016; 28(3):483–490

[33] Raiskila S, Axelin A, Rapeli S, Vasko I, Lehtonen L. Trends in care practices reflecting parental involvement in neonatal care. Early Hum Dev. 2014; 90(12):863–867

[34] Schweitzer M, Aucoin J, Docherty SL, Rice HE, Thompson J, Sullivan DT. Evaluation of a discharge education protocol for pediatric patients with gastrostomy tubes. J Pediatr Health Care. 2014; 28(5):420–428

[35] Sharma N, Sargent J. Overview of the evidence base for family interventions in child psychiatry. Child Adolesc Psychiatr Clin N Am. 2015; 24(3):471–485

[36] Shi M, Xu MY, Liu ZL, et al. Effectiveness of family involvement in newly diagnosed type 2 diabetes patients: a follow-up study. Patient Educ Couns. 2016; 99(5):776–782

[37] Thompson-Hollands J, Edson A, Tompson MC, Comer JS. Family involvement in the psychological treatment of obsessive-compulsive disorder: a meta-analysis. J Fam Psychol. 2014; 28(3):287–298

[38] Tucker JM, Eisenmann JC, Howard K, et al. FitKids360: design, conduct, and outcomes of a stage 2 pediatric obesity program. J Obes. 2014; 2014:370–403

[39] van Wassenaer-Leemhuis AG, Jeukens-Visser M, van Hus JWP, et al. Rethinking preventive post-discharge intervention programmes for very preterm infants and their parents. Dev Med Child Neurol. 2016; 58 Suppl 4:67–73

[40] Young AS, Fristad MA. Family-based interventions for childhood mood disorders. Child Adolesc Psychiatr Clin N Am. 2015; 24(3):517–534

[41] Vahedian-Azimi A, Miller AC, Hajiesmaieli M, et al. Cardiac rehabilitation using the Family-Centered Empowerment Model versus home-based cardiac rehabilitation in patients with myocardial infarction: a randomised controlled trial. Open Heart. 2016; 3(1):e000349

[42] Phillips F, Prezio EA. Wonders & Worries: evaluation of a child centered psychosocial intervention for families who have a parent/primary caregiver with cancer. Psychooncology. 2017; 26(7):1006–1012

[43] Lester P, Liang LJ, Milburn N, et al. Evaluation of a family-centered preventive intervention for military families: parent and child longitudinal outcomes. J Am Acad Child Adolesc Psychiatry. 2016; 55(1):14–24

[44] Deek H, Hamilton S, Brown N, et al. family Project Investigators. Family-centred approaches to healthcare interventions in chronic diseases in adults: a quantitative systematic review. J Adv Nurs. 2016; 72(5):968–979

[45] Gallo KP, Hill LC, Hoagwood KE, Olin SCS. A narrative synthesis of the components of and evidence for patient- and family-centered care. Clin Pediatr (Phila). 2016; 55 (4):333–346

[46] Michie S, Miles J, Weinman J. Patient-centredness in chronic illness: what is it and does it matter? Patient Educ Couns. 2003; 51(3):197–206

[47] Chu SY. Family-centred applied behaviour analysis verbal behaviour intervention for young Taiwanese children with disabilities. Int J Early Years Educ. 2016; 24(1):80–96

[48] Mittal V. Family-centered rounds. Pediatr Clin North Am. 2014; 61(4):663–670

[49] Thompson GA, McFerran KS, Gold C. Family-centred music therapy to promote social engagement in young children with severe autism spectrum disorder: a randomized controlled study. Child Care Health Dev. 2014; 40(6):840–852

[50] Torenholt R, Schwennesen N, Willaing I. Lost in translation—the role of family in interventions among adults with diabetes: a systematic review. Diabet Med. 2014; 31(1):15–23

[51] Bock DE, Robinson T, Seabrook JA, et al. The Health Initiative Program for Kids (HIP Kids): effects of a 1-year multidisciplinary lifestyle intervention on adiposity and quality of life in obese children and adolescents—a longitudinal pilot intervention study. BMC Pediatr. 2014; 14:296

[52] Ansari A, Gershoff E. Parent involvement in head start and children's development: indirect effects through parenting. J Marriage Fam. 2016; 78(2):562–579

[53] Dunst CJ, Trivette CM, Hamby DW. Meta-analysis of family-centered helpgiving practices research. Ment Retard Dev Disabil Res Rev. 2007; 13(4):370–378

[54] Baig AA, Benitez A, Quinn MT, Burnet DL. Family interventions to improve diabetes outcomes for adults. Ann N Y Acad Sci. 2015; 1353(1):89–112

[55] Cooper L, Morrill A, Russell RB, Gooding JS, Miller L, Berns SD. Close to me: enhancing kangaroo care practice for NICU staff and parents. Adv Neonatal Care. 2014; 14(6):410–423

[56] Mataji Amirrood M, Taghdisi MH, Shidfar F, Gohari MR. The impact of training on women's capabilities in modifying their obesity-related dietary behaviors: applying family-centered empowerment model. J Res Health Sci. 2014; 14(1):75–80

[57] Marsh S, Foley LS, Wilks DC, Maddison R. Family-based interventions for reducing sedentary time in youth: a systematic review of randomized controlled trials. Obes Rev. 2014; 15(2):117–133

[58] Nayeri ND, Mohammadi S, Razi SP, Kazemnejad A. Investigating the effects of a family-centered care program on stroke patients' adherence to their therapeutic regimens. Contemp Nurse. 2014; 47(1–2):88–96

[59] Cason-Wilkerson R, Goldberg S, Albright K, Allison M, Haemer M. Factors influencing healthy lifestyle changes: a qualitative look at low-income families engaged in treatment for overweight children. Child Obes. 2015; 11(2):170–176

[60] Fischer RL, Anthony ER, Lalich N, Blue M. Addressing the early childhood mental health needs of young children: evaluating child and family outcomes. J Soc Serv Res. 2014; 40(5):721–737

[61] Woods DT, Catroppa C, Godfrey C, Giallo R, Matthews J, Anderson VA. Challenging behaviours following paediatric acquired brain injury (ABI): the clinical utility for a manualised behavioural intervention programme. Soc Care Neurodisability. 2014; 5(3):145–159

[62] Woods DT, Catroppa C, Godfrey C, Anderson VA. Long-term maintenance of treatment effects following intervention for families with children who have acquired brain injury. Soc Care Neurodisability. 2014; 5(2):70–82

[63] Grzyb MJ, Coo H, Rühland L, Dow K. Views of parents and health-care providers regarding parental presence at bedside rounds in a neonatal intensive care unit. J Perinatol. 2014; 34(2):143–148

[64] Oczkowski SJW, Mazzetti I, Cupido C, Fox-Robichaud AE. The offering of family presence during resuscitation: a systematic review and meta-analysis. J Intensive Care. 2015; 3:41

[65] Wielaert SM, Sage K, Heijenbrok-Kal MH, Van De Sandt-Koenderman MWME. Candidacy for conversation partner training in aphasia: findings from a Dutch implementation study. Aphasiology. 2016; 30(6):699–718

[66] Yeh HY, Ma WF, Huang JL, Hsueh KC, Chiang LC. Evaluating the effectiveness of a family empowerment program on family function and pulmonary function of children with asthma: a randomized control trial. Int J Nurs Stud. 2016; 60:133–144

[67] Cuesta-Barriuso R, Torres-Ortuño A, López-García M, Nieto-Munuera J. Effectiveness of an educational intervention of physiotherapy in parents of children with haemophilia. Haemophilia. 2014; 20(6):866–872

[68] Weis J, Zoffmann V, Egerod I. Enhancing person-centred communication in NICU: a comparative thematic analysis. Nurs Crit Care. 2015; 20(6):287–298

[69] Crespo C, Santos S, Tavares A, Salvador Á. "Care that matters": family-centered care, caregiving burden, and adaptation in parents of children with cancer. Fam Syst Health. 2016; 34(1):31–40

[70] Kuhlthau KA, Bloom S, Van Cleave J, et al. Evidence for family-centered care for children with special health care needs: a systematic review. Acad Pediatr. 2011; 11(2):136–143

[71] Garrouste-Orgeas M, Périer A, Mouricou P, et al. Writing in and reading ICU diaries: qualitative study of families' experience in the ICU. PLoS One. 2014; 9(10):e110146

[72] Mann D. Design, implementation, and early outcome indicators of a new family-integrated neonatal unit. Nurs Womens Health. 2016; 20(2):158–166

[73] Ingram JC, Powell JE, Blair PS, et al. Does family-centred neonatal discharge planning reduce healthcare usage? A before and after study in South West England. BMJ Open. 2016; 6 (3):e010752

[74] Górska S, Forsyth K, Prior S, Irvine L, Haughey P. Family group conferencing in dementia care: an exploration of opportunities and challenges. Int Psychogeriatr. 2016; 28(2):233–246

[75] Kuo DZ, Bird TM, Tilford JM. Associations of family-centered care with health care outcomes for children with special health care needs. Matern Child Health J. 2011; 15(6):794–805

[76] Shulkin D, O'Keefe T, Visconi D, Robinson A, Rooke AS, Neigher W. Eliminating visiting hour restrictions in hospitals. J Healthc Qual. 2014; 36(6):54–57

[77] Dennis BM, Nolan TL, Brown CE, et al. Using a checklist to improve family communication in trauma care. Am Surg. 2016; 82(1):59–64

[78] Salani D. Implementation of shift report at the bedside to promote patient- and family-centered care in a pediatric critical care unit. J Nurses Prof Dev. 2015; 31(2):81–86

[79] Roter D, Hall J. The influence of physician characteristics on communication between the doctor and the patient. In: Roter D, ed. Doctors Talking with Patients. Patients Talking with Doctors. Wesport: Praeger; 2006

[80] Demehri FR, Claflin J, Alameddine M, et al. Surgical baseball cards: improving patient- and family-centered care. J Surg Educ. 2015; 72(6):e267–e273

[81] Hielkema M, De Winter AF, Feddema E, Stewart RE, Reijneveld SA. Impact of a family-centered approach on attunement of care and parents' disclosure of concerns: a quasi-experimental study. J Dev Behav Pediatr. 2014; 35(4):292–300

[82] Dhillon A, Tardini F, Bittner E, Schmidt U, Allain R, Bigatello L. Benefit of using a "bundled" consent for intensive care

unit procedures as part of an early family meeting. J Crit Care. 2014; 29(6):919–922

[83] Desai AD, Popalisky J, Simon TD, Mangione-Smith RM. The effectiveness of family-centered transition processes from hospital settings to home: a review of the literature. Hosp Pediatr. 2015; 5(4):219–231

[84] Gonya J, Martin E, McClead R, Nelin L, Shepherd E. Empowerment programme for parents of extremely premature infants significantly reduced length of stay and readmission rates. Acta Paediatr. 2014; 103(7):727–731

[85] Oshimura JM, Downs SM, Saysana M. Family-centered rounding: can it impact the time of discharge and time of completion of studies at an academic children's hospital? Hosp Pediatr. 2014; 4(4):228–232

[86] Charmel PA, Frampton SB. Building the business case for patient-centered care. Healthc Financ Manage. 2008; 62(3):80–85

[87] Hsieh RL, Hsieh WH, Lee WC. Short-term family-centered workshop for children with developmental delays enhances family functioning and satisfaction: a prospective clinical trial. Medicine (Baltimore). 2016; 95(31):e4200–e4200

[88] Law M, Hanna S, King G, et al. Factors affecting family-centred service delivery for children with disabilities. Child Care Health Dev. 2003; 29(5):357–366

[89] Meyer C, Scarinci N, Ryan B, Hickson L. "This is a partnership between all of us": audiologists' perceptions of family member involvement in hearing rehabilitation. Am J Audiol. 2015; 24(4):536–548

[90] Sugden E, Baker E, Munro N, Williams AL. Involvement of parents in intervention for childhood speech sound disorders: a review of the evidence. Int J Lang Commun Disord. 2016; 51(6):597–625

[91] Tosh R, Arnott W, Scarinci N. Parent-implemented home therapy programmes for speech and language: a systematic review. Int J Lang Commun Disord. 2017; 52(3):253–269

[92] Bright FAS, Kayes NM, Cummins C, Worrall LM, McPherson KM. Co-constructing engagement in stroke rehabilitation: a qualitative study exploring how practitioner engagement can influence patient engagement. Clin Rehabil. 2017; 31 (10):1396–1405

[93] Rosewilliam S, Roskell CA, Pandyan AD. A systematic review and synthesis of the quantitative and qualitative evidence behind patient-centred goal setting in stroke rehabilitation. Clin Rehabil. 2011; 25(6):501–514

[94] McKean K, Phillips B, Thompson A. A family-centred model of care in paediatric speech–language pathology. Int J Speech-Language Pathol. 2012; 14(3):235–246

[95] Thomas-Stonell N, Oddson B, Robertson B, Rosenbaum P. Predicted and observed outcomes in preschool children following speech and language treatment: parent and clinician perspectives. J Commun Disord. 2009; 42(1):29–42

[96] Jones M, Onslow M, Packman A, et al. Randomised controlled trial of the Lidcombe programme of early stuttering intervention. BMJ. 2005; 331(7518):659

[97] Ciccone N, Hennessey N, Stokes SF. Community-based early intervention for language delay: a preliminary investigation. Int J Lang Commun Disord. 2012; 47(4):467–470

[98] Kong NY, Carta JJ. Responsive interaction interventions for children with or at risk for developmental delays. Top Early Child Spec Educ. 2013; 33(1):4–17

[99] Lawler K, Taylor NF, Shields N. Outcomes after caregiver-provided speech and language or other allied health ther-

apy: a systematic review. Arch Phys Med Rehabil. 2013; 94 (6):1139–1160

[100] Roberts MY, Kaiser AP. The effectiveness of parent-implemented language interventions: a meta-analysis. Am J Speech Lang Pathol. 2011; 20(3):180–199

[101] Roberts MY, Kaiser AP. Assessing the effects of a parent-implemented language intervention for children with language impairments using empirical benchmarks: a pilot study. J Speech Lang Hear Res. 2012; 55(6):1655–1670

[102] Simmons-Mackie N, Raymer A, Cherney LR. Communication partner training in aphasia: an updated systematic review. Arch Phys Med Rehabil. 2016; 97(12):2202–2221.e8

[103] Law J, Garrett Z, Nye C. Speech and language therapy interventions for children with primary speech and language delay or disorder. Cochrane Developmental, Psychosocial and Learning Problems Group. 2003(3)

[104] Hawkins DB. Effectiveness of counseling-based adult group aural rehabilitation programs: a systematic review of the evidence. J Am Acad Audiol. 2005; 16(7):485–493

[105] Heydebrand G, Mauze E, Tye-Murray N, Binzer S, Skinner M. The efficacy of a structured group therapy intervention in improving communication and coping skills for adult cochlear implant recipients. Int J Audiol. 2005; 44(5):272–280

[106] Chisolm TH, Arnold M. Evidence about the effectiveness of aural rehabilitation programs for adults. In: Wong L, Hickson L, eds. Evidence-Based Practice in Audiology: Evaluating Interventions for Children and Adults with Hearing Impairment. San Diego, CA: Plural Publishing, Inc.; 2012:237–266

[107] Keen D, Meadan H, Brady NC, Halle JW. Prelinguistic and minimally verbal communicators on the autism spectrum. Singapore: Springer; 2016

[108] Lang R, Machalicek W, Rispoli M, Regester A. Training parents to implement communication interventions for children with autism spectrum disorders (ASD): a systematic review. Evid Based Commun Assess Interv. 2009; 3(3):174–190

[109] Eggenberger E, Heimerl K, Bennett MI. Communication skills training in dementia care: a systematic review of effectiveness, training content, and didactic methods in different care settings. Int Psychogeriatr. 2013; 25(3):345–358

[110] Lucía Habanec O, Kelly-Campbell RJ. Outcomes of group audiological rehabilitation for unaided adults with hearing impairment and their significant others. Am J Audiol. 2015; 24(1):40–52

[111] Johansson B, Carlson M, Ostberg P, Sonnander K. A multiple-case study of a family-orientated intervention practice in the early rehabilitation phase of persons with aphasia. Aphasiology. 2013; 27(2):201–226

[112] National Health and Medical Research Council. Statement on consumer and community involvement in health and medical research: Consumers Health Forum of Australia. 2016; https://www.nhmrc.gov.au/guidelines-publications/s01. Accessed November 12, 2018

[113] McKenzie A, Hanley R. Planning for consumer and community participation in health and medical research: a practical guide for health and medical researchers. 2014; http://www.involvingpeopleinresearch.org.au/find-out-more/our-resources/the-purple-book 2014 Accessed November 12, 2018

[114] O'Brien MJ, Whitaker RC. The role of community-based participatory research to inform local health policy: a case study. J Gen Intern Med. 2011; 26(12):1498–1501

Chapter 2

Getting Ready to be a Patient- and Family-Centered Clinician

2 Getting Ready to be a Patient- and Family-Centered Clinician

Caitlin Barr

Abstract

A key factor influencing the successful implementation of patient- and family-centered care is the clinician himself or herself. With the appropriate skills, traits, and attributes, the clinician can foster the development of an effective therapeutic relationship with the patient and his or her family, encourage patients and families to be the drivers of their care, and ensure their management is holistic, taking into consideration the patient and family's biopsychosocial needs, preferences, and context. The way a clinician communicates with patients and families reflects his or her underlying attitudes, values, and priorities, and therefore can make patients and families feel understood, cared for, respected, and listened to. In order to develop these patient- and family-centered skills, it is important that clinicians regularly partake in reflective practice. Patient- and family-centered communication skills improve with reflection and practice, much like all skills health professional acquire. This chapter discusses the range of communication skills that patient- and family-centered speech–language pathologists and audiologists must practice, including nonverbal communication, questioning, listening, and empathy.

Keywords: patient-centered care, family-centered care, patient- and family-centered communication, empathy, reflection

Learning Objectives

In this chapter student speech–language pathologists and audiologists will learn the following:
1. How to undertake clinical reflection using formal reflection tools.
2. The role of communication in enabling the patient–family–clinician relationship.
3. How to identify and describe the four key aspects of clinician communication for patient- and family-centered care.
4. How to maximize their communication skills, including nonverbal communication, listening, questioning, and empathy.
5. The importance of self-care in being a patient- and family-centered clinician.

2.1 Introduction to Getting Ready to be a Patient- and Family-Centered Clinician

"At the end of the day people won't remember what you said or did, they will remember how you made them feel."

(Maya Angelou)

This quote certainly rings true in the context of health care and for health professionals. Clinicians can make patients and families feel understood, cared for, respected, listened to or in contrast, it can also make them feel distant, a nuisance, or an unimportant person. The way a clinician communicates, both verbally and nonverbally, reflects his or her underlying attitudes, values, and priorities, along with the attitudes, values, and priorities of the clinician's workplace. Such attitudes, values, and priorities are considered environmental factors in the International Classification of Functioning, Disability and Health (ICF).[1] That is, the way a clinician communicates with patients and families is a mediating factor in how patients and families experience their health conditions. At all times, you, as the speech–language pathologist or audiologist, should remain respectful in how you communicate with patients and their families. Respectful behaviors and the respectful use of language are key to developing effective patient–family–clinician therapeutic relationships. CanChild has developed a helpful fact sheet for using respectful behaviors and language, and we encourage you to refer to this and remain mindful of the key messages when interacting with patients and their family. Click here to access the factsheet: https://www.canchild.ca/system/tenon/assets/attachments/000/001/274/original/FCS9.pdf

2.2 The Patient–Family–Clinician Therapeutic Relationship

In Chapter 1 of this book, you were introduced to the conceptual model of patient- and family-centered care (PFCC) (▶ Fig. 2.1). The first core

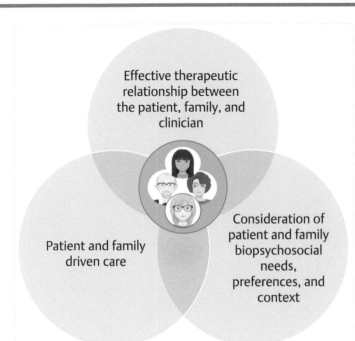

Fig. 2.1 Integrated model of patient- and family-centered care.

Effective therapeutic relationship between the patient, family, and clinician

Patient and family driven care

Consideration of patient and family biopsychosocial needs, preferences, and context

principle of PFCC was the development of an effective therapeutic relationship between the patient, family, and clinician. As speech–language pathologists and audiologists, you will often have the opportunity to develop long-term therapeutic relationships with patients and families, and therefore it is essential to understand how you can build and successfully maintain these relationships.[2,3] Even if you work in an acute hospital setting where decisions are made quickly, and you may not necessarily go on to have a long-term therapeutic relationship with patients and their families, having the skills to quickly develop a trusting relationship is key to practicing PFCC.

Relationships with patients and families are developed through effective clinician communication. This was highlighted in the systematic review conducted by Scholl et al[4] (as discussed in Chapter 1), where the most pertinent enabler of PFCC was clinician–patient communication. Similarly, much research has emphasized the fundamental role of communication skills in providing patient-centered care.[5]

What are your current thoughts on your role and values as a speech–language pathologist or audiologist? These thoughts are likely to change as you progress through the book. Therefore, let's capture your preferences right now, before we go any further, so you can look back and compare them down the track. Go ahead and complete the Patient Practitioner Orientation Scale (▶ Fig. 2.2). There are no right or wrong answers!

Once you have completed the questionnaire, follow the marking guide and work out your scores. You will end up with a Total Score, a Sharing Score, and a Caring Score. Please note before scoring yourself that three of the questions require reverse scoring (items 9, 13, 17). To calculate your score for Subscale 1: SHARING, add all scores from questions 1 to 9 and divide by 9. To calculate your score for Subscale 2: CARING, add all scores from questions 10 to 18 and divide by 9. Finally, to calculate your TOTAL score, add all scores from all questions and divide by 18. Higher scores indicate higher levels of patient-centeredness.

Patient practitioner oriented scale items

Score
1 = Strongly agree
2 = Somewhat agree
3 = Agree
4 = Disagree
5 = Somewhat disagree
6 = Strongly disagree

1. The audiologist/SLP is the one who should decide what gets talked about during an appointment.

2. Although health care is less personal these days, this is a small price to pay for therapeutic advances.

3. The most important part of the standard appointment is the test.

4. It is often best for clients if they do not have the full explanation of their test results.

5. Clients should rely on their audiologist/SLP's knowledge and not try to find out about their conditions on their own.

6. When audiologists/SLPs ask a lot of questions about a client's background, they are prying too much into personal matters.

7. If audiologists/SLPs are truly good at diagnosis and treatment, the way they relate to clients is not that important.

8. Many clients continue asking questions even though they are not learning anything new.

9. Clients should be treated as if they were partners with the audiologist/SLP, equal in power and status.

10. Clients generally want reassurance rather than information about their audiologic condition.

11. If an audiologist/SLP's primary tools are being open and warm, the audiologist/SLP will not have a lot of success.

12. When clients disagree with their audiologist/SLP, this is a sign that the audiologist/SLP does not have the client's respect and trust.

13. A management plan cannot succeed if it is in conflict with a client's lifestyle or values.

14. Most clients want to get in and out of the audiologist/SLP's office as quickly as possible.

15. The client must always be aware that the audiologist/SLP is in charge.

16. It is not that important to know a client's culture and background in order to treat the client's audiologic condition.

17. Humour is a major ingredient in the audiologist/SLP's management of the client.

18. When clients look up audiologic information on their own, this usually confuses more than it helps.

Fig. 2.2 Modified patient-practitioner orientation scale (PPOS).[6]

2.3 Evidence for the Importance of Communication Knowledge and Skills

Substantial research evidence reveals that no matter how knowledgeable a clinician is, if he or she is not a skilled communicator, knowledge transfer will be lost, and patients and families will not receive the information they need to make important health care decisions. This notion was clearly reflected in the opening quote for this chapter. From previous research, we know that there is a strong, positive relationship between a clinician's communication and interaction skills, and outcomes such as treatment adherence,[7,8] patient satisfaction,[9] and health outcomes.[10,11] If communication with a clinician is poor, patients will report feeling that they are not being listened to, cared about, or provided with enough information.[5]

For communication to be patient- and family-centered, speech–language pathologists and audiologists need to consider their own internal barriers to providing PFCC and how to continually improve their own communication; be cognizant of patients' and family members' experiences and emotions; and, have the ability to adapt communication so that all patients and families receive information in a clear, unbiased, and straightforward manner that is sensitive and meaningful to them. This chapter will first explore the importance of reflective practice in being a patient- and family-centered clinician and how this applies to clinician behavior change. Following this, communication will be explored across four key skill areas: (1) nonverbal communication; (2) exploration (questioning); (3) listening; and (4) empathy (the importance of working with your patient's and family's emotions).

Interesting Fact

Did you know that patient–family–clinician communication is the *most commonly performed* clinical "procedure" across a clinician's professional lifetime? Despite this, evidence suggests that clinicians typically invest very little time in reflecting on and updating their communication skills or improving their ability to communicate.

Student Activity 2.2: What Makes a Patient- and Family-Centered Clinician?

In pairs or small groups, brainstorm, then create a mind map of the skills, traits, and attitudes that you believe make a speech–language pathologist or audiologist patient- and family-centered. Start with a circle in the middle of a large page of paper, or on a white board.

Skills, traits, and attitudes of a PFCC speech–language pathologist or audiologist

After you have finished your brainstorming activity, group together the skills, traits, and attitudes that are similar or complementary. Once your skills, traits, and attitudes are grouped, highlight the ones that relate to communication specifically.

2.4 A Reflective Clinician Is a Patient- and Family-Centered Clinician

As clinicians, we are often encouraged to start keeping the end in mind; that is, to set goals that we want to work toward or set outcomes we want to achieve. In the case of becoming a patient- and family-centered clinician, the truth is, there is no end! A truly patient- and family-centered clinician sets on a path where the main principle is that of continual improvement, where each clinical encounter and moment of communication helps you to learn, shape, and fine-tune your communication skills.

Communication is more than being able to "do a task." In fact, it is arguably more difficult than much of the other clinical work we do as speech–language pathologists and audiologists as there are no hard-and-fast rules for all scenarios. Patient- and family-centered communication involves being self-aware (i.e., being able to understand and appropriately manage one's own reactions and beliefs); flexible and adaptable in understanding what others are saying without making assumptions of "knowing"; responsive to others' needs, personalities, cultures, and preferences; and to be able to respond in a sensitive way. That is, a clinician needs to have a good sense of his or her own emotional reactions, comfort zones, and communication abilities. This can be achieved through reflective practice.

So, what is reflection? Reflection is an important life skill (see TEDx presentation by James Schmidt https://youtu.be/G1bgdwC_m-Y), but one that also applies specifically to health professionals. Reflection is a process by which professionals, through their own experiences as well as others, ultimately gain new insights about themselves and their practice. A reflective practitioner is one who uses reflection as a tool for revisiting experiences and critically appraising these experiences in order to learn from and shape future clinical encounters.[12]

Reflective practice involves two separate but linked processes: (1) reflection-in-action (i.e., the ability to think and act on your feet); and (2) reflection-on-action (i.e., the ability to analyze a situation and the reasons for and consequences of your actions).[13] In order to reflect-in-action and on-action, you will need skills in self-awareness, critical thinking, and mindful practice. Self-awareness refers to the cognitive ability to think, feel, sense, and know through intuition, and to evaluate this knowledge to develop understanding, whereas critical thinking involves being able to identify and challenge one's own assumptions.[14] Lastly, mindful practice involves attending to one's own physical and mental processes during clinical tasks in a nonjudgmental way.[15]

2.4.1 Frameworks and Tools for Reflection

There are a number of different ways you can reflect on your clinical practice and fine-tune your reflective practice skills. A clinical supervisor may ask you to verbally reflect after a clinical encounter, or you might choose to write a reflective journal or blog, video or audio record a consultation, engage in peer discussion, or role play. Reflective writing is the most common way of formalizing reflective practice. This allows clinicians to make their reflections concrete and observable to others, and offers a professional development opportunity. There are also structured tools that you can use and two of the most popular are Kolb's learning cycle[16] and Gibbs' reflective cycle. Kolb's learning cycle relates

to learning generally, whereas Gibbs' reflective cycle (▶ Fig. 2.3) builds on Kolb's framework and provides structure appropriate to health care.

Student Activity 2.3: Practice Reflective Practice

Think of a recent communication encounter with a patient or family member that did not go as well as you would have liked. Using Gibbs' reflective cycle (▶ Fig. 2.3), reflect on this clinical encounter. Once you have finished, swap your reflection with a peer. Discuss your experiences of completing Gibb's reflective cycle.

2.5 Key Areas in Which Speech–Language Pathologists and Audiologists Should Reflect: Internal Barriers to Providing PFCC

As discussed in Chapter 1, a consistent finding in health care research is a mismatch between the agreed importance of providing quality, evidence-based PFCC, and what happens in actual clinical care. This mismatch highlights how hard it can be to implement PFCC in practice and reminds us how important it is to reflect on the barriers to providing PFCC. One way to conceptualize the barriers that clinicians can face in providing PFCC is to consider theories of behavior change and one of the theories that is particularly useful in this context is the Behavior Change Wheel.[18] In the context of becoming a patient- and family-centered clinician, the Behavior Change Wheel considers the need for clinicians to have the **Capability** (skills, knowledge, and confidence), **Opportunity** (time, resources, and support), and **Motivation** (values and incentives) to behave in a particular way.[18–20] An example of a capability barrier is that clinicians may feel they do not have the skills and confidence to have difficult conversations with patients and families (e.g., delivering bad news, or seeing people cry).[21] An example of an opportunity barrier would be having appointment times that are too short to allow PFCC.[5] Finally, a motivation barrier could be that the values and culture of the organization in which the clinician works do not support PFCC.[22,23] In fact, it has been reported that student health professionals show concern that their patient-centeredness might decline once in the workplace.[24] Perhaps you share this concern too?

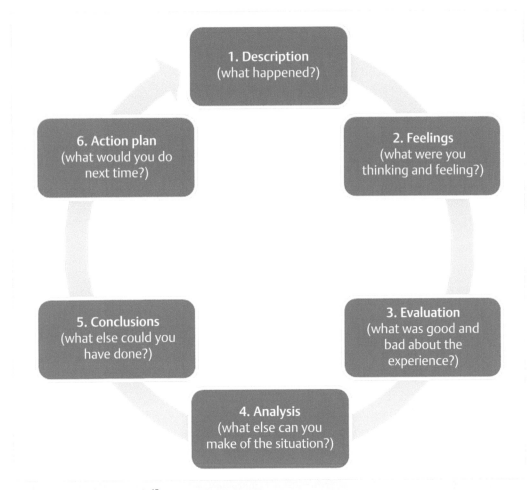

Fig. 2.3 Gibbs' reflective cycle.[17]

It is worthwhile taking a minute now, and periodically throughout your studies and career to reflect on your barriers to providing PFCC. You can very simply ask yourself: To what extent are the following things impacting my ability to be a patient- and family-centered speech–language pathologist or audiologist?
• *Capability (skills, knowledge, and confidence).*
• *Opportunity (time, resources, and support within the organization or peers).*
• *Motivation (values, attitudes, and incentives).*

Once you have reflected (formally or informally), you can go about putting a plan in place to overcome or work around the barriers. It may also shape what you look for in a workplace and how you work with others. Remember to keep a focus on your role in caring for patients and their families.

2.6 Communication Skills of a Patient- and Family-Centered Speech–Language Pathologist and Audiologist

The following section will delve into the four communication skill areas required to be a patient- and family-centered clinician, including: (1) nonverbal communication; (2) exploration; (3) listening; and (4) empathy (▶ Fig. 2.4). Each of these skills does not come easy and requires commitment from you, not only now as you are

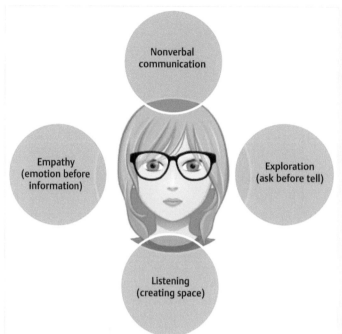

Fig. 2.4 Four key communication skills for speech–language pathologists and audiologists.

training to be a speech–language pathologist or audiologist, but also after you graduate as you continue to hone your communication skills. Take a moment now to view **Video 2.1** to hear from Bettina Turnball, an experienced audiologist, about "Top Tips" for getting ready to be a patient- and family-centered clinician.

2.6.1 Nonverbal Communication

Studies exploring the impact of clinician communication on patient outcomes have found that a combination of verbal and nonverbal communication is important; however, information about the best mix of these two elements is less clear.[25] Interestingly though, observational studies have reported that patients respond more strongly to clinicians' nonverbal messages than their verbal messages or, at least, are very aware of a clinician's nonverbal communication style. For example, in a study of recorded consultations between general practitioners and patients, when receiving diagnostic information, patients reported being affected by the clinicians' body language rather than the diagnostic information itself. Importantly, if you're working with patients or family who have a hearing loss or who are deaf, or who have receptive language difficulties, you need to be

particularly sensitive to your nonverbal communication skills. People who have difficulty accessing or understanding auditory input, no matter what degree, are likely to rely more heavily on nonverbal communication. Therefore, it is widely advocated that speech–language pathologists and audiologists should pay at least as much attention to nonverbal communication skills as verbal skills.[25-27]

What is nonverbal communication? Broadly speaking, nonverbal communication is communication without, or extends beyond, the use of spoken language. Nonverbal communication can be described in five categories:

1. Proxemics: The physical environment in which communication is occurring (e.g., placement of chairs and desk; height difference of chairs) (see Chapter 3).
2. Movement and body: Kinesics (flow of movement), gestures (any body movement including head nods), posture, body orientation and leaning, and haptics (touch).
3. Facial expressions.
4. Eye contact.
5. Paralanguage: Including verbal elements (voice quality, emotion, speaking style), and prosodic features (intonation and stress), influenced by the use of pauses, interruptions, and cutoffs.

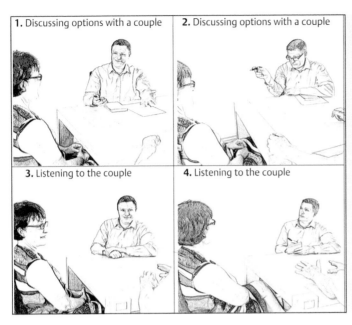

1. Discussing options with a couple

2. Discussing options with a couple

3. Listening to the couple

4. Listening to the couple

Fig. 2.5 Comparison of nonverbal communication.

It is widely reported that clinicians' nonverbal communication represents their underlying attitudes and beliefs. For example, see the image above (▶ Fig. 2.5). In both drawings, the clinician says the same words to the patient and their family member, but what differs is how the clinician is sitting and his or her body language. The images on the left hand side of the figure show patient- and family-centered communication behaviors whereby the clinician is open and engaged, looking directly at the patient and the family member while discussing options and listening to their response. Conversely, in the images on the right hand side of the figure, the clinician is not displaying patient- and family-centered communication, rather, exhibiting a sense of control in the situation and ignoring the family members' communication attempts.

Student Activity 2.5: Interpreting Nonverbal Communication

The purpose of this activity is to pay close attention to the messages clinicians and patients give using nonverbal communication. For this activity, you'll need access to the volume control on your computer or audiovisual (AV) device.

1. Play the Case History video "Pediatric Case History #1" (**Video 2.2**) with the volume at a comfortable level, but look away from the screen or turn the screen off so that you cannot see the interaction between the clinician and the patient.
2. Answer the questions provided in ▶ Fig. 2.6, Part 1.
3. Replay the video and watch the interaction, but this time with the volume off (i.e., observing the nonverbal communication).
4. Answer the questions provided in ▶ Fig. 2.6, Part 2.
5. Answer the questions provided in ▶ Fig. 2.6, Part 3.
6. Complete the same exercise with the video "Pediatric Case History #2" (**Video 2.3**).

After completing these exercises, discuss the Part 3 questions in a small group: what, if any, differences did you note between the verbal and nonverbal communication? If you did note any differences, which of the messages do you think were truer to the person's true message? Were the verbal or nonverbal messages more likely to contain emotion? Why do you think this was?

Part 1: Listening but not seeing—verbal communication

1. What is your sense of how well this interaction is going? Explain what is it that gives you this sense.
2. To what extent do both parties sound comfortable and involved?
3. What do you notice in the clinician's voice and language?
4. What do you notice in the mother's voice and language?

Part 2: Seeing but not hearing—nonverbal communication

1. What is your sense of how well this interaction is going? Explain what is it that gives you this sense.
2. To what extent do both parties look comfortable and involved?
3. What do you notice in the clinician's body language?
4. What do you notice in the mother's body language?

Part 3: Put it all together

1. Do the verbal and nonverbal communication align in this video?
2. Of the verbal and nonverbal communication, which do you think represents how the participants are feeling most accurately?
3. Were the verbal or nonverbal messages more likely to contain emotion?
4. How, if at all, might you change the communication in this interaction to optimise it?

Fig. 2.6 Reflection questions about nonverbal communication.

2.6.2 Exploration (Ask before You Tell)

As a patient- and family-centered clinician, one of your core principles is to consider the patient and family's biopsychosocial needs, preferences, and contexts. Obtaining this information requires well-developed skills in asking questions and managing interpersonal dynamics. Here, the process of gaining insight into patients' and families' biopsychosocial contexts is termed "exploration" quite on purpose. Think of your clinical interactions as journeys where you may have some idea of the end you're aiming for, as will your patient, but the path in between requires a sense of adventure and non-judgmental curiosity. Your exploration should encapsulate all areas of the ICF, from body functions and structures, to activities and participation, and contextual factors. Chapter 5 will elaborate on tools you might be able to use to elicit information from patients and families; however, the following section will focus on the underlying skills of exploring.

Say you find yourself in an initial consultation with Shane and Lorna, whom you met in Chapter 1 of this book. Shane has been recently forced to retire, due to a deterioration in his functioning because of Parkinson's disease. How do you go about exploring the biopsychosocial needs, preferences, and contexts of Shane and Lorna? Well, you have to ask! The skill being of course, the *way* you ask the question.

Open- and closed-ended questions: You are likely familiar with the terms "open-ended" and "closed-ended" questions, but you may not have thought about how they should be used in health care interactions.

A closed-ended question is often defined as one where the answer is "yes" or "no." However, for the purposes of health care communication, closed-ended questions are defined as questions which can be answered with a single word or phrase, for example: How old are you? Where do you live? Closed-ended questions are set up by the first word in a question (e.g., do, would, are, will, have…), and any other question can be turned into a closed-ended question by adding tag questions to the end (e.g., isn't it? don't you?). Remembering this will remind you that it is important to start your question correctly, and to be careful that a well-phrased open-ended question does not unintentionally become a closed-ended question.

Closed-ended questions are useful and important in particular instances because of the following:
• They give you facts.
• They are quick and easy to answer.
• They maintain clinicians' control of the conversation.

Closed-ended questions are therefore most useful for checking understanding, clarifying, and summarizing (e.g., Have I understood this correctly? Is this what you meant when you said…?), and therefore play an important role in health care communication.

Open-ended questions can be defined as requesting long-form information or an elaboration from the patient or family member being questioned. Open-ended questions are important and useful because of the following:

- They ask the person being questioned to think and reflect.
- They will elicit opinions and feelings.
- They hand over control of the conversation to the person being questioned.

For these reasons, open-ended questions are ideally used to explore a patient and family member's needs, preferences, and context, to specifically explore feelings and facts, and, to allow people to feel like they are being listened to and cared for. Open-ended questions usually start with "what, why, how, describe." As a speech–language pathologist or audiologist, using open-ended questions can be challenging and scary as they require you to hand over control to the patient and/or family members. However, a well-placed and considered open-ended question can elicit a plethora of important information and will save you time in the end by not having to request specific information using closed-ended questions.

On a side note, you may have heard of a third type of question—the leading question! Leading questions are framed in such a way that the respondent is led to answer in a particular way, or to avoid a particular answer, that is, the respondent is led to answer in the way that they feel is the "right" answer, rather than the truthful one. For this reason, leading questions are to be avoided.

Read the following questions and (1) identify which questions are leading; then (2) try to rewrite these questions so that they are no longer leading. For example, "So you're having trouble with your hearing?" could be rewritten as "Tell me more about what is happening with your hearing."

- So, you've never experienced this before?
- There's no history of this condition in your family, is there?
- You don't expect that you'll get back to being 100%, do you?
- When are you planning on doing something to improve this?
- How badly does this impact you?

Principles of Exploration through Asking Questions

Open with open: The first question asked by a speech–language pathologist or audiologist as part of the clinical consultation is critical to setting up the feeling, power balance, and agenda for the consultation and relationship and therefore requires careful planning and consideration. While many clinicians will have asked the social question "how has your day been?" on the walk between the waiting room and the clinical room, this is actually a good time to practice open-ended questioning, with the first clinical question then marking a transition to the health care interaction. So, what should the ideal opening question be? Ideally, it should be open ended, not too confronting, show that you want to share the agenda setting, and can be followed up on easily. For example, instead of asking "Can you share with me how you feel about your diagnosis?." You could ask "How do you feel about your diagnosis?"

Top Tip

To maximize the likelihood of successfully opening your conversation with a patient and family, have *two* open-ended questions ready to go. Many clinicians find that if they have just one question, and the patient or family isn't ready or comfortable elaborating, the conversation becomes stuck and the clinician falls quickly into a closed-ended questioning style, just like in the example below.

Case Example: Version 1

Clinician: Shane, tell me what the last few weeks have been like since you retired?
Shane: Terrible
Clinician: Oh, I'm sorry to hear that. And have your symptoms changed over that time?

Case Example: Version 2

Clinician: Shane, tell me what the last few weeks have been like since you retired?
Shane: Terrible
Clinician: Oh, I'm sorry to hear that. It's certainly a substantial change for you. Can you tell me more about what you've been experiencing?

The use of open-ended and closed-ended opening questions can be observed in the Pediatric Case History videos (**Video 2.2** and **Video 2.3**). Watch these videos and observe how open-ended and closed-ended questions can lead to different types of interactions and to different types of information being shared.

As a speech–language pathologist or audiologist in training, planning your opening question can set you up for an effective consultation, but you may not get it right every time. If you have an experience where it doesn't work for you, or where it works particularly well, use your reflective practice skills to explore this further. Let's have a go at putting this into practice.

Student Activity 2.7: Practicing Exploration

In pairs or groups of three, nominate each person to the role of either (1) asking the questions; (2) responding to the questions; and (3) observing (if possible). Have the observer set a timer for 5 minutes. The questioner should decide on a topic to talk about that is of interest to the person being questioned (e.g., sport, art, and travel).

There are two parts to this activity:

Part 1: The questioner should first ask a closed-ended question, and then follow up with mostly closed-ended questions. The questioner should take notes of the information gained. The person being questioned should only respond to the questions being asked. The observer should take note of the overall feeling of the interaction and the quality of the rapport being developed.

Part 2: The questioner should ask an open-ended question to begin with, and then follow up with open-ended questions. The questioner should take notes of the information gained. The person being questioned should respond only to the questions being asked. The observer should take note of the overall feeling of the interaction and the quality of the rapport being developed.

Take it in turns to fulfill each role.

Get feedback on exploration

Discuss in your group both scenarios in relation to the amount of information obtained, the quality of information obtained, and the impact on rapport building.

Reflect on exploration

After your group discussion, consider how comfortable you felt in both scenarios and what this means for your own clinical practice. If you found it hard asking open-ended questions, this could be an area for future professional development.

Follow-up and clarify: A second principle of exploration is that the information provided by patients and families is appropriately followed up and clarified to ensure that you have the whole and correct picture. If the patient and/or family brings up an important point that may not fit with the current conversation, be sure to note this, mentally or physically, so that you can follow it up. You may flag that you will follow it up while keeping the conversation on track by saying "that's an interesting point, let's come back to that shortly." This ensures that the person who made the point feels listened to and valued.

Clarification is important because it ensures you have heard and understood the patient and family correctly. Clarification can take the form of quick checks, for example, sorry, did you say? or when you say X, do you mean Y? Clarification takes place within running conversations and often uses a closed-ended question. Be careful about how you clarify and avoid interruptions where possible.

Summarize and check: Summarizing and checking goes beyond clarification and typically takes place at the end of a speaker's turn or conversation. For example, Lorna may have just told you all about how she has been altering her participation to ensure she is available to take care of her husband, Shane. After the interaction, you should summarize the key points and how you understood them, checking back with her that you have understood her facts and feelings correctly. Summarizing and checking requires the use of both open- and closed-ended questions, along with a reassurance or acknowledgement that you are taking the floor, for example:

"Thank you for sharing that with me. From what you have shared, I understand that this has impacted you both significantly. Lorna, have I understood it correctly that you've stopped going to all your social activities at this point in time? Is that correct? Or are there some activities that you can still do now?"

It is important to summarize and check before moving on to a new topic for exploration.

Feelings and facts: One of the key differences between open- and closed-ended questions is that open-ended questions can elicit both feelings and facts, whereas closed-ended questions elicit facts alone. It is widely understood that people experience their health and functioning practically and emotionally and so health professionals must understand and address both aspects. The timing of questioning is important here. For example, as a speech–language pathologist or audiologist, you should start a consultation with open-ended questions, but unless you have already built a relationship with the patient and family, questions with emotional content should be used later in a consultation and ideally as a follow-up. For example, you could ask Lorna and Shane:

"You've shared with me a great deal about the practical impact this has had on you both. I'm also interested in the impact this has had on you emotionally. Tell me more about that."

The importance of asking and responding to feelings is further discussed in the section below on Empathy.

2.6.3 Listening (Creating Space)

Listening is a skill we learn at an early age and is often taken for granted. Perhaps you have been told by friends that you're a good listener or you've thought that of someone else? What does it mean to be a good listener? When learning to become a patient- and family-centered clinician, you need to hone your listening skills to include active listening, empathetic listening, reflective listening, and creation of space. In this context, listening extends beyond the act of hearing, to interpretation of information and feelings, and setting up an environment where people are comfortable sharing personal information.

Types of listening: Passive listening can be defined as simply hearing information and is a one-way process. In contrast, active listening occurs when the listener is fully engaged with, and reacts to, the speaker and communication is taking place in a two-way process. That is, the listener, although not contributing content to the conversation, is present and contributing in paraverbal ways (e.g., mmm, I see). If the clinician has actively listened to the patient and family, the clinician is then able to check if he or she has correctly understood the patient and family's thoughts and feelings by offering his or her interpretation of the message back to the patient and family. This process is called reflective listening.

In counseling and other talk-based therapies, active listening is considered as a fundamental skill. More specifically, empathetic listening, or entering the privately perceived world of another, highlights the importance of not only just being active in listening, but also active in responding to the speaker. Not surprisingly then, active and empathetic listening take a lot

of effort on the part of the clinician. Active listening requires a combination of both verbal and nonverbal communication skills. Essentially, a clinician who is an active listener is the one who does the following:

- Pays attention and is not distracted (this includes taking notes or using the computer).
- Regularly acknowledges the patient's or family's message and encourages them to continue.
- Provides a combination of verbal and nonverbal feedback to convey attention and response to the message.
- Defers judgement or opinion.
- Does not take the conversation floor until the patient or family is finished.

Interruptions and pauses are important markers of active listening whereby interruptions suggest that the clinician is wanting to regain control and is not listening (nor interested) in the patient's or family's message, whereas pauses provide an environment where the patient and family feel there is space for them to elaborate, and that the clinician is interested. Active listening is more difficult than what it may seem. For example, in a study where 63 audiology consultations with adult patients were video recorded, and where communication was observed, it was found that many audiologists did not engage in active listening at the beginning of the consultation, with 62% of opening questions being closed-ended in nature and the clinician interrupting patient talk, on average, after 21.3 seconds.[28]

Case Example

Speech–language pathologist: Emily, the results from today's assessment suggest that things are improving with your vocal nodules; this is great news. However, you did say when you came in that things aren't going well at the moment, can you share with me some more about this?

Emily: Oh, no, it's fine—you're right, my voice is improving…[here the clinician could agree and move on; alternatively, the clinician decides to create space by acknowledging but encouraging Emily to continue talking].
Speech–language pathologist: Yes, your voice is improving; however, I'm interested if there are other things concerning you, or what questions you have…?
Emily: (pauses) Well, I guess you could say I've lost a bit of confidence…

Speech–language pathologist: mmhmm (nods).
Emily: (pauses) I'm starting to dislike playing with
my band and I don't like talking in front of people at
University which is making things a bit awkward…
Hugh thinks I'm withdrawing and is starting to get
frustrated when I don't want to go out to parties
with him…
Speech–language pathologist: (pauses, and when
Emily doesn't add anything further…) Emily, that
sounds like you're having a really tough time.
[consultation continues]

You can see that there are a number of crucial points where, as a clinician, you can decide to close down a conversation, or create space by using a combination of "exploring techniques" and "creating space." By creating space, you are able to obtain important psychosocial information from your patient that will help you provide high-quality care. In this example, the speech–language pathologist is able to work with Emily to make a decision regarding further voice therapy with goals relating to confidence, not just good vocal hygiene and practices, along with discussing techniques to overcome embarrassment when Emily's voice quality changes with nerves. Thus, the clinician addresses Emily's individual needs thoroughly. The clinician is also able to talk about whether her band mates and lecturers might need some information about how they can support her.

Watch the video "Working with Parental Concerns" (**Video 2.4**) and think about which aspects of this video show signs of active listening and passive listening, and the consequences of these behaviors.

Now that you have a better understanding of active listening and why it is important, read the excerpt in the box (A Word from a Clinical Expert: Creating a "Listening Space") by Dr. Kris English, an audiologist, who describes the therapeutic nature of active listening.

Practicing active and reflective listening: Listening skills can be improved by practicing, getting feedback, and reflecting. Have a go at the following "Student Activity 2.9" and then be sure to ask for feedback from your educators whenever you're seeing patients as well.

Practice listening

In pairs or groups of three, set up a role play where one person is the listener, another the talker, and the third an observer (if possible).

The listener should start by asking the talker a question about a general topic (e.g., holidays, weather, news events) and then have a conversation for about 5 minutes and the listener should listen in the way that comes most naturally to them. The observer is encouraged to take notes—refer to the template in ▶ Fig. 2.7.

Get feedback on listening

Before providing feedback, the observer (or listener if in a pair) should first ask the talker and listener for their reflections on the interaction— what went well and what could have been improved? After this, the observer can talk through their written feedback. When providing feedback, be descriptive (not judgmental) and constructive. Give the talker and listener an opportunity to ask questions.

Repeat the activity so that each person in the pair or group of three has a turn at being the "listener."

Reflect on listening

After everyone has had a turn at being the "listener," refer to ▶ Fig. 2.8 and reflect on your experiences of active listening.

2.6.4 Empathy (Being with Emotions)

"The purpose of the doctor is to: cure sometimes,
relieve often and comfort always"

(Socrates)

So far, we have learned that your communication skills are a powerful part of your clinical toolbox. Of all the research that has explored the impact of communication on patient and family outcomes, many have reported that empathy, or response to emotion, is a critical component of patient–family–clinician communication. Why is working with emotions so important? Seeking and responding to emotions, specifically, being empathetic and showing empathy, facilitates trust,[30] leads to higher-quality disclosure of information,[31] improves treatment adherence,[32] and is therapeutic; that is, empathy helps patients and families in its own right.[31]

1. What was the opening question and was it open ended, closed ended, or leading?
2. In your opinion, did the listener demonstrate passive or active listening? Why do you think this? *For example, did they interject to ask additional questions?* *Did they encourage the other to continue talking by using 'uhuh' or 'yes, I see' type statements?*
3. What went well in this interaction? Did the listener get sufficient information from the talker? Did the conversation end too quickly?
4. Did the talker appear comfortable when they were talking?
5. Did the listener appear genuinely interested in the talker?

Fig. 2.7 Practicing listening: questions for the observer.

1. Description: what happened?
2. Feelings: what were you thinking and feeling?
3. Evaluation: what was good and bad about the experience?
4. Analysis: what sense can you make of the situation?
5. Conclusion: what else could you have done?
6. Action plan: if the situation arose again, what would you do?

Fig. 2.8 Applying Gibbs' reflective model to your listening practice.

A Word from a Clinical Expert: Creating a "Listening Space"

Dr. Kris English, Audiologist, United States

Recently I was in line at a doctor's office, behind a departing patient. He was scheduling a set of follow-up appointments, and while the desk person scanned calendar options, the patient made three attempts to connect with her. He commented on the weather; he mentioned a local sports team; and he expressly thanked her for carefully attending to this task. For unknown reasons, the scheduler did not make eye contact, respond to his remarks, or confirm the final arrangements. Instead, she handed him a piece of paper, looked past him and said, "Next!"

I will never know why the scheduler tuned out this patient, but I will also never forget the expression on his face when he turned and left: disappointed, lonely, and hurt. He walked away with less human contact than he was hoping for, and it clearly mattered.

We are probably saying to ourselves, "How awful—I would never do that!" We don't see ourselves as nonlisteners; however, we may not have given much thought to what listening actually entails. Until we do, we could unintentionally fall into similar nonresponse patterns. Specifically, we must be able to distinguish between everyday listening (the minimum we can do, although the scheduler did not) and therapeutic listening, an advanced and essential skill for all clinicians.

As the name implies, everyday listening is part of the routine give-and-take in ordinary conversation. We've been doing it all our lives, and it involves minimal attention, energy, and courtesy. The challenge is this: how do we know when a conversation is not everyday? Sometimes it's obvious ("I just spent the morning at a child's funeral service"). Often, though, an ordinary conversation masks a more serious concern; for example, "I've heard children are more likely to be born with a disability when the mother works right up to the due date." Many times, our patients and their families have far more on their minds than small talk. There are countless kinds of troubles, but for now take a moment and imagine one life challenge patients and families might be facing. (If you are drawing a blank, consult with an educator.) Now, how would a patient or family member extend an invitation to be heard and understood? As mentioned, it could be a direct appeal ("funeral"), but it often starts with a comment that indirectly alludes to a concern. It's a risk: Will the request for a listener be perceived?

Let's assume we do perceive the invitation, be it verbal, nonverbal, or by metamessage. When we respond with openness and acceptance, an amazing thing happens: We create a kind of space that didn't exist before, a trusting interpersonal space where fears are unburdened, catharsis occurs, insights develop, isolation diminishes. As the speaker communicates, the listener sets aside agendas, refrains from giving advice, tries to empathize, and actively turns the moment over to the speaker.

We can describe this selfless act as therapeutic listening because of known positive outcomes. When we create opportunities for patients and families to verbalize their fears, express their worries, and talk through options, doubts, and possibilities, they either find their way to a solution, or they (and we) realize that the situation needs help from a professional counselor. The listener realizes therapeutic benefit as well, perhaps from new insight into human nature, a clarification to an old assumption, or a boost in emotional intelligence.

On the topic of listening, Palmer[29] offers this observation: "Virtually all professionals have been deformed by the myth that we serve our clients best by taking up all the space with our hard-won omniscience" (p. 132). Our educational programs do not intentionally try to "deform" us with myths; it's just the nature of professional training. Our career-long challenge is to overcome that myth, resist the tendency to dominate "all the space," and put our "hard-won omniscience" to the side. Once we understand the power of sharing emotional space with another, we will never again say in bewilderment, "All I did was listen." We will know exactly how listening helped.

Think back to the families you were introduced to in Chapter 1: Each case showed that individuals and families have unique experiences that go beyond the biomedical cause of their condition. In the ICF, this is highlighted by the interrelationship between the lived experiences of communication impairment (i.e., activity limitations and participation restrictions) and contextual factors (i.e., environmental and personal factors). In all cases, irrespective of the condition and experiences, a commonality is that each person involved will have an emotional reaction to his or her circumstance, and this in turn will influence how he or she seeks help, copes with changes, and moves forward with treatment or rehabilitation.

Emotions are known to be influential drivers of ability to understand and remember information, decision making, and ability to change behavior.[33] While there has been substantial research exploring the biological and psychological influences of emotions (such as stress) on patients' health behaviors,[34] less has focused on how clinicians can optimally work with patients and families who are experiencing a myriad of emotions. In your role as a speech–language pathologist or audiologist, you may be providing diagnoses to families, and giving news about expected outcomes, prognoses, or progress that will be emotional. In your work, you will need to provide emotional support as your patients may not yet have created their own support network; families may adjust at different times and patients may have differences in their emotional literacy (how they can express how they feel). Ultimately, you will find yourself in a vital role of acknowledging, supporting, and guiding your patients and families through their psychosocial experiences.[33,35–38]

What do emotions look like and what will influence emotions? Patients and families are likely to experience some common emotions. As speech–language pathologists and audiologists, it is important to consider what these emotions might look like or sound like, and they might differ across diverse cultures, races, genders, and ages.

- Fear (what does this mean for me and my family?).
- Anger (why me?).
- Sadness or disappointment (sense of loss).
- Shame or guilt (this is my fault).
- Relief (this isn't as bad as I expected).

The most common strategy for working with emotions is to be empathetic and show empathy. Empathy, in a clinical context, can be defined as the clinician's ability to understand patients' and families' emotions, and can be felt, shown, and imparted in many ways. A challenge for clinicians is that many professional bodies recognize the importance of empathy, yet advocate that clinicians perform empathy rather than feel it.[31] For example, one professional association for doctors in the United States defines empathy as "the act of correctly acknowledging the emotional state of another without experiencing that state oneself."[31] Others argue that a health professional cannot be empathetic without sharing a feeling with the patient or family. That is, it is more than acknowledging the presence of emotion.

Empathy: What is it?

What empathy is:
- Involves being moved by another's experience.

What empathy isn't:
- Empathy is not feeling sorry, upset, or sad for a patient or a family. You may have heard, or said yourself, "I feel sorry for ....". This is what is known as *sympathy*, which, in a clinical context, reinforces the power imbalance between the patient, family, and clinician and creates distance between patients' and families' experiences, and the clinician.
- Detached concern. This concept suggests that it is sufficient for a clinician to know that a patient is feeling anxious, but not have to know what anxiety might feel like. That is, detached concern says that a clinician can label a patient's or family's feelings in the absence of connecting with the actual feeling.

Student Activity 2.10: Empathy versus Sympathy

"Empathy fuels connection; sympathy fuels disconnection"

(Brené Brown)

This quote summarizes one of the biggest misnomers in a clinician's communication toolbox. Take a look at Brené Brown's RSA animated talk on empathy on YouTube (https://www.youtube.com/watch?v=KZBTYViDPlQ). Then, reflect on (1) what the main points were; (2) how this relates to being a speech–language pathologist or audiologist; and (3) how empathy would differ from sympathy in your professional work?

How do I be empathetic? Given that empathy is needed to provide PFCC, speech–language pathologists and audiologists need to learn to empathize effectively with patients and their families. It is therefore important to know that it is possible to learn or be taught how to be empathetic[39]; however, empathy cannot be taught in a textbook!

Empathy is not just knowledge, it is an attitude or a task. It is a process that encompasses effective (feelings), cognitive (thinking), and behavioral (doing) tasks. That is, simply feeling empathy and not communicating it will not be effective, nor will communicating an empathic response without being authentic about it. Underlying empathy are several attitudes and beliefs. Professionals need patience, curiosity, and a willingness to open up in order to feel connected with a patient and family and their experience.[40] To be empathetic and show genuine empathy, remember the importance of the patient–family–clinician relationship and consider the following general guidelines[41]:

- **You are a listener and supporter, but not a therapist.** A sensitive conversation about emotions will benefit your patients, but you do not need to resolve or move your patients or families past their emotions. This requires you to have a comfort in "sitting with emotions," that is, be present, no matter how uncomfortable, and resist the need to make your patient feel better or feel worried that you can't fix the problem for them.
- **Use your listening skills.** Be on the lookout for emotional language or body language and ensure you then explore and listen to this. Make eye contact, move closer, and use the patient's name to reassure that you are present with them.
- **Use emotional language and reflect back the feelings they are showing.** Do not be afraid to name the emotion your patients or families are showing (like the examples provided above; "I see that this is making you sad"). Naming emotions allows the patient to feel heard and helps him or her to understand his or her own emotions. Talking about emotions is important in normalizing the experience and moves away from hiding or not dealing with emotions as they are experienced.
- **Resist the "righting reflex."** Speech–language pathologists and audiologists care about their patients' well-being, want people to feel/cope

better, and are good problem solvers. While these are important traits of health professionals, when it comes to emotions, it is important to remember that it isn't your role to fix the problem or minimize or erase emotions. A specific example of this is that when a patient or family is describing a scenario, decisions, or ways of thinking, which do not align with your ideals, or that you know how to overcome, the unconscious temptation is to jump in and try to fix or correct the situation; this is the righting reflex. To best facilitate patients' and families' management of their emotions, it is important to resist this temptation and instead, encourage the patients or families to come to decisions themselves. This concept is explained in detail in the counseling strategy called "motivational interviewing,"[42] which utilizes the skills described here, in a particular structure (see Interesting Fact below and article review by McFarlane[43]).

Interesting Fact: Motivational Interviewing Explained

Motivational interviewing is a process guided by four principles[43,44]:
- **Express empathy** through the use of reflective listening.
- **Develop discrepancy** (i.e., awareness of discrepancies between a patient and family member's current behaviors and their goals/values) through careful clinical guidance.
- **Roll with resistance** by demonstrating respect for the patient and family member and highlighting their autonomy in decision making processes.
- **Support self-efficacy** by reassuring patients and family members that they're capable of change.

Four key skills have also been identified for the implementation of motivational interviewing, including the use of open questions, affirmations, reflections, and summaries.[44]

Read the excerpt on next page from Katie Ekberg that illustrates how empathy can be used and how opportunities for empathy can be missed in health consultations. For a more detailed exploration of this excerpt, refer to the following paper.[35]

Katie Ekberg, Psychologist, Australia

Patients often raise emotional talk during health care appointments, including within speech–language pathology and audiology appointments. Various aspects of the patient's life may come up during appointments that carry a negative emotional stance (e.g., worry, sadness, disappointment, or fear). An important aspect of patient- and family-centered care is that patients' emotional talk is responded to with a caring and empathic nature by the health care professional. These responses facilitate a good therapeutic relationship. Below is a real-life example of an empathic response from an audiologist within an assessment appointment with an adult patient. The example comes from the history-taking phase of the appointment. In the transcript below, A = audiologist, and P = patient. Nonverbal actions that occur across the participants' turns are marked with a * for the audiologist and + for the patient.

Example 1

```
 1 A: Um:: (0.4) *any family history of hearing loss?*
              *leans forward, looking at C——–*
 2 P: Ah: (.) [my mother had a hearing- ] *well [she-] she was- lived-*
    A:                                  *starts typing————–*
 3 A:     [Just parents or siblings.] [Yeah]
 4 P: + oh died just last year but-= +
       + places hands up to head, wipes forehead +
 5 A: *=I'm sorry to [hear that.]*
        *Stops typing, looks at C, leans forward*
 6 P:      [She lived] 'til ninety four so .hhh
 7 A: *[ > That's < a good innings.]*
        *Looking at C————–*
 8 P: [and she had a hearing] aid yeah.
 9    *(1.1)*
    A: *Nods, starts typing again*
10 P: In oh prob'ly (0.7)
11 A: *Just later in life [though? ]*
        *Looks up at C————–*
12 P:     [Probably] about the eighties [yeah.]
13 A:                           [Okay.]
```

   In line 1 of this fragment, the audiologist asks the patient about any family history of hearing loss. This is a standard history-taking question that is asked of all patients within the information-gathering phase of audiology appointments. In line 2, the patient begins to respond to this question by talking about his mother's hearing loss. His turn here is full of hesitations and restarts, and at line 4, he eventually discloses that his mother died "just last year." The types of hesitations across the patient's turns are often seen when someone has something difficult or challenging to say. The audiologist, at line 5 (bolded), responds quickly with an empathic response to this news: "I'm sorry to hear that." This commiseration statement orients to the affective stance of the patient's prior turn. It displays "other attentiveness" from the audiologist, rather than just pursuing his own agenda of gathering information about the patient's hearing loss. In this way, the audiologist establishes rapport with the patient by showing listening and understanding of the patient's response. The audiologist's nonverbal actions also consist of stopping typing, looking up at the patient, and leaning forward. These actions, again, show the patient that the audiologist's attention is focused on him, and what they are saying. This turn from the audiologist does not take a lot of time but performs an important function in building a relationship with the patient. The audiologist then keeps his or her attention on the patient until he finishes speaking.

   The next example comes from another real-life, audiology assessment appointment, with a different audiologist and adult patient. This example demonstrates a "missed opportunity" for empathy where the audiologist does not respond or orient to the emotional nature of the patient's talk.

Continued ▶

Example 2

1 A: Is there any family history of hearing loss (0.4) that you know of?

2   (0.2)

3 P: + No:: my parents are both dead.=They've been dead since I was

      + Periodically looks down at table throughout turn———

4   seventeen so +

          ——— +

5 A: **Okay.**

6   (0.5)

7 A: Have you ever um been exposed to loud noises in any:: (.) like jobs

8   that you did or hob[bies] that you had?

9 P: [No.]

In this fragment, the audiologist, at line 1, asks the same history-taking question to the patient as seen above. In lines 3 and 4, the patient provides an elongated "no::" and discloses that both her parents have been dead since she was a teenager. Throughout her turn she glances down at the table as well as up at the audiologist. So again here, the patient has produced a turn that has a negative emotional stance and, therefore, invites an empathic response from the audiologist. However, in this case, the audiologist responds with a minimal acknowledgement "Okay" (bolded) and then moves on to her next history-taking question about exposure to loud noises. She does not orient to the emotional nature of the patient's turn. This response from the audiologist thus marks a missed opportunity to display empathy to the patient. Rather, the audiologist focuses on her agenda of gathering information about the patient's hearing history.

Student Activity 2.11: Identifying Opportunities for Empathy

Another example of an opportunity where empathy was needed can be observed in the video "Relationship Building" (**Video 2.5**). Watch this video and look out for the clinician's opportunities for empathy, and discuss with your peers whether these opportunities were used optimally, and if not, what could have been done differently.

Students and teachers of communication for speech–language pathologists and audiologists are encouraged to explore online resources such as http://empathetics.com/ to learn more about empathy, and are encouraged to practice it daily!

Student Activity 2.12: How Well Do You Communicate with Clients?

Take a copy of the CARE questionnaire (▶ Fig. 2.9) with you to your next clinical placement. With your supervisor or educator's permission, give the questionnaire to a number of your patients and ask them to complete it as a way of assisting you as you continue to develop your clinical communication skills. Then, reflect on your results:

• What did the results tell you?
• Are you surprised by these results?
• How will the results impact your future communication?

Please rate the following statements about today's consultation How good was the practitioner at…..	Score 1 = Poor 2 = Fair 3 = Good 4 = Very good 5 = Excellent
1. Making you feel at ease (*being friendly and warm towards you, treating you with respect; not cold or abrupt*)	
2. Letting you tell you "Story" (*giving you time to fully describe your illness in you own words; not interrupting or diverting you*)	
3. Really listening (*paying close attention to what you were saying; not looking at the notes or computer as you were talking*)	
4. Being interested in you as a whole person (*asking/knowing relevant details about you life, you situation; not treating you as 'just a number'*)	
5. Making you feel at ease (*being friendly and warm towards you, treating you with respect; not cold or abrupt*)	
6. Showing care and compassion (*seeming genuinely concerned, connecting with you on a human level; not being indifferent or 'detached'*)	
7. Being positive (*having a positive approach and a positive attitude; being honest but not negative about you problems*)	
8. Explaining things clearly (*fully answering your questions, explaining clearly, giving you adequate information; not being vague*)	
9. Helping you take control (*exploring with you what you can do to improve your health yourself; encouraging rather than lecturing you*)	
10. Making a plan of action with you (*discussing the options, involving you in decision as much as you want to be involved; not ignoring you views*)	

Fig. 2.9 Consultation and relational empathy (CARE).[45] (Available for free download from www.caremeasure.org).

2.7 A Final Note: Clinician Self-Care

Much of this book is focused on how to optimally care for patients and families who are experiencing a change in communication functioning. You may be surprised to hear that it is now time to talk about the importance of caring for yourself.

In this chapter, we have discussed the importance of building meaningful therapeutic relationships with patients and families, exploring and understanding people as a whole, and being an empathetic clinician. These skills require you to personally invest in your work at a physical and emotional level. Without considering how this will affect you over the course of your career, or immediately, when confronted with a challenging or upsetting scenario, you may run the risk of "burning out." Clinician self-care is widely recognized as an essential part of being a patient- and family-centered clinician, and numerous resources are becoming available. It is beyond the scope of this book to explore the techniques directly; however, the authors encourage speech–language pathologists and audiologists to invest time in exploring the concepts of mindfulness and avoiding burnout.

2.7.1 Case Example

The clinician who works with Andrew, and his parents, Miranda and Flynn invests heavily in ensuring that Miranda and Flynn are coping with the significant changes in their life since Andrew was diagnosed with autism spectrum disorder. This involves extensive discussion about both practical and emotional aspects of their well-being. For example, since quitting work to be part of Andrew's early intervention, Miranda seems to have low mood and gets teary in most consultations. The clinician finds these sessions draining emotionally and is starting to feel less able to be as compassionate as is needed; that is, the clinician fears that he is burning out. To counter this concern, the clinician seeks out time with a mentor in his organization to debrief on this case, and specifically discuss the impact it is having on him as the clinician. With the mentor's advice, the clinician schedules in an extra 15 minutes after consultations with this family where he writes down the impact it is having on him, as a way of removing the weight from his shoulders. The clinician also takes 5 minutes to get fresh air before commencing the next consultation.

After implementing these simple self-care strategies, Miranda notes at the next consultation that the clinician seems very "present," which she greatly appreciates; and the clinician feels able to work closely with this family long into the future.

2.8 Summary

To ensure that you're ready to start the long journey of being a patient- and family-centered clinician across your career working with people who have communication disability and their families, you need to ensure you have the skills, traits, and attributes of a great communicator. Being a reflective practitioner is central to being a patient- and family-centered clinician, and this chapter contains a number of suggestions and practical tools for how to do this on a regular basis. Communication skills that will allow you to be a patient- and family-centered clinician are also described in this chapter: being attentive to nonverbal as well as verbal communication, exploring the perspectives of patients and families, using open-ended questions, creating space, actively listening, following up and clarifying, and last, but by no means least, being empathetic. These skills will set you up to provide high-quality PFCC to your patients, families, and yourself.

2.9 Reflections

Please respond to the following reflection questions in your PFCC journal:

1. What are the three dimensions of the Behavior Change Wheel important to consider when implementing PFCC in clinical practice?
2. What are the five categories of nonverbal communication in a clinical setting?
3. Consider a recent clinical encounter in speech–language pathology or audiology where you detected emotion in what was conveyed by the patient and/or the family. What was the emotion and how did you respond? How did you show empathy in the way you responded?

References

[1] World Health Organization. ICF, International Classification of Functioning, Disability and Health. Geneva: World Health Organization; 2001

[2] Worrall L, Davidson B, Hersh DJ, et al. The evidence for relationship-centred practice in aphasia rehabilitation. J Interact Res Commun Disord. 2010; 1(2): 277-300

[3] Grenness C, Hickson L, Laplante-Lévesque A, Davidson B. Patient-centred care: a review for rehabilitative audiologists. Int J Audiol. 2014; 53 Suppl 1:S60–S67

[4] Scholl I, Zill JM, Härter M, Dirmaier J. An integrative model of patient-centeredness—a systematic review and concept analysis. PLoS One. 2014; 9(9):e107828

[5] Levinson W, Lesser CS, Epstein RM. Developing physician communication skills for patient-centered care. Health Aff (Millwood). 2010; 29(7):1310–1318

[6] Laplante-Lévesque A, Hickson L, Grenness C. An Australian survey of audiologists' preferences for patient-centredness. Int J Audiol. 2014; 53 Suppl 1:S76–S82

[7] Bolkan CR, Bonner LM, Campbell DG, et al. Family involvement, medication adherence, and depression outcomes among patients in veterans affairs primary care. Psychiatr Serv. 2013; 64(5):472–478

[8] Nayeri ND, Mohammadi S, Razi SP, Kazemnejad A. Investigating the effects of a family-centered care program on stroke patients' adherence to their therapeutic regimens. Contemp Nurse. 2014; 47(1–2):88–96

[9] Wanzer MB, Booth-Butterfield M, Gruber K. Perceptions of health care providers' communication: relationships between patient-centered communication and satisfaction. Health Commun. 2004; 16(3):363–383

[10] Mead N, Bower P. Patient-centred consultations and outcomes in primary care: a review of the literature. Patient Educ Couns. 2002; 48(1):51–61

[11] Bertakis KD, Azari R. Determinants and outcomes of patient-centered care. Patient Educ Couns. 2011; 85(1):46–52

[12] Mann K, Gordon J, MacLeod A. Reflection and reflective practice in health professions education: a systematic review. Adv Health Sci Educ Theory Pract. 2009; 14(4):595–621

[13] Joyce-McCoach J, Smith K. A teaching model for health professionals learning reflective practice. Procedia Soc Behav Sci. 2016; 228:265–271

[14] Finlay L. Reflecting on 'Reflective practice'. PBLB paper. 2008;52

[15] Epstein RM. Mindful practice in action (I): Technical competence, evidence-based medicine, and relationship-centered care. Fam Syst Health. 2003; 21(1):1–9

[16] Kolb DA. Learning styles inventory. The Power of the 2 2 Matrix. 2000:267

[17] Gibbs G. Learning by Doing: A guide to Teaching and Learning Methods. Oxford Centre for Staff and Learning Development; 2013

[18] Michie S, van Stralen MM, West R. The behaviour change wheel: a new method for characterising and designing behaviour change interventions. Implement Sci. 2011; 6(1):42

[19] Michie S, West MA. Managing people and performance: an evidence based framework applied to health service organizations. Int J Manag Rev. 2004; 5/6(2):91–111

[20] Légaré F, Ratté S, Gravel K, Graham ID. Barriers and facilitators to implementing shared decision-making in clinical practice: update of a systematic review of health professionals' perceptions. Patient Educ Couns. 2008; 73(3):526–535

[21] Meyer EC, Sellers DE, Browning DM, McGuffie K, Solomon MZ, Truog RD. Difficult conversations: improving communication skills and relational abilities in health care. Pediatr Crit Care Med. 2009; 10(3):352–359

[22] Luxford K, Safran DG, Delbanco T. Promoting patient-centered care: a qualitative study of facilitators and barriers in healthcare organizations with a reputation for improving the patient experience. Int J Qual Health Care. 2011; 23(5):510–515

[23] Gillespie R, Florin D, Gillam S. How is patient-centred care understood by the clinical, managerial and lay stakeholders

responsible for promoting this agenda? Health Expect. 2004; 7(2):142–148

[24] Bombeke K, Symons L, Debaene L, De Winter B, Schol S, Van Royen P. Help, I'm losing patient-centredness! Experiences of medical students and their teachers. Med Educ. 2010; 44(7): 662–673

[25] Little P, White P, Kelly J, et al. Verbal and non-verbal behaviour and patient perception of communication in primary care: an observational study. Br J Gen Pract. 2015; 65(635):e357–e365

[26] D'Agostino TA, Bylund CL. Nonverbal accommodation in health care communication. Health Commun. 2014; 29(6): 563–573

[27] Roter DL, Frankel RM, Hall JA, Sluyter D. The expression of emotion through nonverbal behavior in medical visits. Mechanisms and outcomes. J Gen Intern Med. 2006; 21 Suppl 1:S28–S34

[28] Grenness C, Hickson L, Laplante-Lévesque A, Meyer C, Davidson B. Communication patterns in audiologic rehabilitation history-taking: audiologists, patients, and their companions. Ear Hear. 2015; 36(2):191–204

[29] Palmer PJ. The courage to teach. San Francisco, CA: Jossey-Bass; 1998

[30] Charon R. The patient-physician relationship. Narrative medicine: a model for empathy, reflection, profession, and trust. JAMA. 2001; 286(15):1897–1902

[31] Halpern J. What is clinical empathy? J Gen Intern Med. 2003; 18(8):670–674

[32] Hojat M, Louis DZ, Maxwell K, Markham F, Wender R, Gonnella JS. Patient perceptions of physician empathy, satisfaction with physician, interpersonal trust, and compliance. Int J Med Educ. 2010; 1:83–87

[33] Singh G, Barr C, Montano J, English K, Russo F, Launer S. The impact of engaging in emotion-based conversations with patients and their families. The Hearing Review. 2017; 24(5):30–32

[34] Ferrer RA, Mendes WB. Emotion, health decision making, and health behaviour. Psychol Health. 2018; 33(1):1–16

[35] Ekberg K, Grenness C, Hickson L. Addressing patients' psychosocial concerns regarding hearing aids within audiology appointments for older adults. Am J Audiol. 2014; 23(3):337–350

[36] Sarno MT. Aphasia rehabilitation: psychosocial and ethical considerations. Aphasiology. 1993; 7(4):321–334

[37] Cruice M, Worrall L, Hickson L, Murison R. Finding a focus for quality of life with aphasia: Social and emotional health, and psychological well-being. Aphasiology. 2003; 17(4):333–353

[38] McAllister J, Collier J, Shepstone L. The impact of adolescent stuttering and other speech problems on psychological well-being in adulthood: evidence from a birth cohort study. Int J Lang Commun Disord. 2013; 48(4):458–468

[39] Fine VK, Therrien ME. Empathy in the doctor-patient relationship: skill training for medical students. J Med Educ. 1977; 52(9):752–757

[40] Larson EB, Yao X. Clinical empathy as emotional labor in the patient-physician relationship. JAMA. 2005; 293(9):1100–1106

[41] Buchman M, McCain GR. After the Diagnosis: How Patients React and How to Help them Cope. 1st ed. Delmar Cengage Learning; New York; 2010

[42] Rollnick S, Miller WR, Butler CC, Aloia MS. Motivational Interviewing in Health Care: Helping Patients Change Behavior. New York; Taylor & Francis; 2008

[43] McFarlane LA. Motivational interviewing: practical strategies for speech–language pathologists and audiologists. Can J Speech-Language Pathol Audiol. 2012; 36(1):8–17

[44] Miller WR, Rollnick S. Motivational Interviewing: Preparing People for Change. 2nd ed. New York, NY: Guildford Press; 2002

[45] Mercer SW, Maxwell M, Heaney D, Watt GC. The consultation and relational empathy (CARE) measure: development and preliminary validation and reliability of an empathy-based consultation process measure. Fam Pract. 2004; 21(6):699–705

Chapter 3

Getting the Environment Ready for Patient- and Family-Centered Care

3 Getting the Environment Ready for Patient- and Family-Centered Care

Nerina Scarinci, Carly Meyer

Abstract

Within the World Health Organization's International Classification of Functioning, Disability and Health (ICF framework), environmental factors are considered to play a key role in how a patient- and his or her family experience a health condition. These environmental factors could be physical, social, or attitudinal in nature, or may refer to the systems and policies of a health system. Social and attitudinal factors are particularly important when considering the implementation of patient- and family-centered care in speech–language pathology and audiology, as are the health services, systems, and policies. This chapter will expand on the role clinicians play in ensuring that physical spaces and the social context are conducive to the implementation of patient- and family-centered care. Within the physical environment, this chapter considers the physical design and setup of the clinical environment, and products and technology for both communication and education. Within the social context, this chapter considers the role of support and relationships as well as the attitudes of family, friends, and acquaintances. This chapter then describes the importance of creating a patient- and family-centered culture within health services, and the important role of professionals at all levels of the organization in this process.

Keywords: patient-centered care, family-centered care, environmental factors, products and technology, attitudes, health services

Learning Objectives

In this chapter, student speech–language pathologists and audiologists will learn the following:

1. The importance of the physical and social environment for patients and their families, including relationships and attitudes.
2. The environmental factors in the International Classification of Functioning, Disability, and Health (ICF) that influence the experience of communication disability for patients and their families.
3. How to prepare the physical clinical environment (including furniture choice and placement, décor and design, and personal effects) to be patient- and family-centered.

4. How to include general assistive technology and specific communication assistive technology in speech–language pathology and audiology practice.
5. How to develop accessible written information for patients with communication disability and their families.
6. What it takes to make an organization patient- and family-centered.

3.1 Introduction to Getting the Environment Ready for Patient- and Family-Centered Care

In Chapter 1, you were introduced to the World Health Organisation's International Classification of Functioning, Disability and Health (ICF).[1] Within the ICF, environmental factors refer to the physical, social, and attitudinal environment in which people live and conduct their lives.[1] This chapter will expand beyond the role you play in the delivery of PFCC to include other aspects of the environment: the physical space, social context, attitudes of other people in the patient's life, and health services, systems, and policies. Physical environmental factors that are particularly relevant to the provision of PFCC include the physical design and set-up of the clinical environment; and products and technology for both communication and education. Within the social context, the role of support and relationships as well as the attitudes of family, friends, and acquaintances will be discussed. Lastly, we will focus on how to enhance the patient- and family-centered culture of speech–language pathology and audiology workplaces.

3.2 Physical Environment

3.2.1 Setting Up the Physical Environment of the Clinical Room

Standard clinical consultation rooms are traditionally very clinician-centered and typically lack the design needed for effective patient, family, and

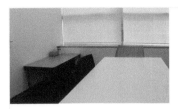
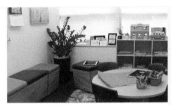
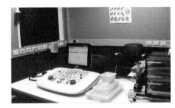
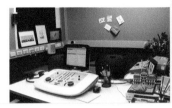

Fig. 3.1 Before and after photos of standard clinical environments versus patient- and family-centered environments.

clinician communication. The images in ▶ Fig. 3.1 highlight some of the key differences between standard clinical rooms and rooms which have been physically adapted to be more patient- and family-centered. These images provide the impetus for the following student activity.

Who doesn't love a "spot the difference" exercise? Above are a series of photos that show a typical clinical room versus a room which has been adapted to be more patient- and family-centered (▶ Fig. 3.1). Without referring to the information that follows in this chapter, identify five differences between the typical clinical rooms on the left and the PFCC rooms on the right and reflect on how these differences might make a patient and his or her family feel.

To see just how easy it is to make a standard clinical room more patient- and family-centered, take a look at two videos we have prepared, one in the context of a pediatric speech–language pathology consultation room (**Video 3.1**), and the other in the context of an adult audiology consultation room (**Video 3.2**).

Why does one space feel more inviting than the other? It turns out that it is not just personal preferences, but rather, there is a body of literature that supports the need to consider the design of

clinical spaces to enhance patient and family member experiences of health services. For example, when you viewed the images of typical clinical rooms versus rooms which have been adapted to be more patient- and family-centered, hopefully one of the first things you noticed was the improved overall ambiance of the spaces, which has known benefits for the patient-family-clinician interaction.[2] The ICF includes codes for various environmental factors, and those that relate to the physical environment specifically, which can be barriers or facilitators to PFCC, are summarized in ▶ Fig. 3.2.[1]

3.2.2 Furniture Choice and Placement

In **Videos 3.1** and **3.2** there was a change in the choice and placement of furniture around the room to accommodate all individuals who would like to attend appointments, in order to promote PFCC. Notably, in the adult example, the chair at the rear of the room was moved next to the patient's chair to promote active family member involvement. In the pediatric example, the large rectangular table was replaced with a round child-sized table, which has been found to reduce fear and anxiety in children.[3] A child-sized bookcase filled with age-appropriate books, toys, and games was also incorporated into the space to provide important play opportunities and to assist the children so that they feel more comfortable and confident in an unfamiliar clinical environment.[3] A play mat was added to the space to encourage floor

Code	Definition	Examples in speech pathology and audiology
e 150 Design, constructions, and building products and technology of buildings for public use		
e1508 Design, construction, and building products and technology of buildings for public use, other specified		• Setting up the physical environment of the clinical room • Furniture choice, placement and style • Decor and design • Personal effects
e125 Products and technology for communication		
e1250 General products and technology for communication	Equipment, products, and technologies used by people in activities of sending and receiving information	• Optical and auditory devices • Audio recorders and receivers • Video conferencing equipment • Telephone devices • Internet • Email
e1251 Assistive products and technology for communication	Adapted or specifically designed equipment, products, and technologies that assist people to send and receive information	• Glasses and contact lenses • Cochlear implants, hearing aids, FM systems • Voice prostheses, communication boards
e 130 Products and technology for education		
e1300 General products and technology for education	Equipment, products, processes, methods and technology used for acquisition of knowledge	• Books • Manuals • Educational toys • Information provided in a range of formats • Universal best practice guidelines for written health information
	Adapted and specifically designed equipment, products, processes, methods and technology used for acquisition of knowledge	• Personalised and individualised treatment regimes • Aphasia friendly guidelines • Adapted materials for people from disadvantaged backgrounds and culturally and linguistically diverse backgrounds

Fig. 3.2 Relevant physical environmental factors related to products and technology and design for patient- and family-centered speech pathology and audiology.

time between the child, family, and clinician in order to engage the pediatric patient in the session and resemble a naturalistic play interaction between a parent and child.

> **Helpful Tip**
>
> Although the clinician will always have an important role in providing therapeutic materials within the clinical space, another consideration for promoting PFCC is to encourage children to bring their own toys or games from home to share with the clinician. To learn other helpful tips for setting up the clinical environment to be more patient- and family-centered for young children and their parents, take a moment to watch Kylie Webb, a speech–language pathologist, set up her clinic room (**Video 3.3**).

As discussed in Chapter 1, a core component of PFCC is the need for an effective therapeutic relationship between the patient, family, and clinician built on trust and mutual respect for one another's strengths and expertise.[4] In order to develop such a therapeutic relationship, clinicians must promote an equal partnership between themselves, the patient, and the family. It may only be a subtle message, but the type of furnishings you place in your clinic rooms plays a role in the balance of power and influence in therapeutic relationships.[5] For example, different sized chairs can infer a power imbalance between patients, families, and clinicians[5] and different sized desks can influence intended patient self-disclosure.[6] In **Videos 3.1** and **3.2**, bench seating was used in place of individual chairs to create a more open and balanced environment. One thing to keep in mind, however, is that bench seating may not always be appropriate given the physical limitations of some patients and family members, and as such, alternate seating should be readily available (e.g., stable chair not on wheels with arm rests).

In the same videos, a separate space was created to hold important clinical conversations with patients and families, for example, for case history taking, goal setting, information sharing, and decision making. This space was purposefully created away from the clinical working area, as holding these discussions across a desk with equipment serving as a physical barrier between the patient, family, and clinician does not foster relationship building and patient- and family-driven care.[5] We acknowledge, however, that there will be times

when you will need to share information with patients and families over the computer, and research suggests that providing patients with clear access to the computer monitor results in patients experiencing increased clinician information sharing, and more time spent engaging in conversations about the information.[7]

We are well aware that as a speech–language pathologist or audiologist, you may have no control over the size of your clinical space or chosen furnishings, but as patients have a general preference for spaciousness,[6] you could consider minimizing the amount of furniture or clutter you have in your consultation room and advocate for flexible furnishings and equipment, which can be tailored to the needs of patients and families.[6]

3.2.3 Décor and Design

In addition to furniture choice and placement, another important consideration for creating a PFCC clinical space is color choice, with research highlighting the important role of color in creating happy, motivating clinical spaces.[3] Specifically, there is some literature supporting the use of cool colors such as blue and green in promoting calmness and relaxation[8] and specifically, in decreasing blood pressure and pulse rate in patients,[9] while pink and yellow have been found to promote feelings of enjoyment and cheerfulness.[8] Interestingly, the color red has been associated with feelings of depression and tiredness,[8] and can lead to unconscious avoidance[10] and reduced performance on cognitive tasks requiring mental manipulation and flexibility.[11] The inclusion of greenery is another important consideration, with literature showing that exposure to greenery can reduce stress and anxiety and improve the overall health care experience.[2,3,12,13] Along these same lines is the consideration of the value of aromatherapy within the clinical space, which has been found to significantly reduce anxiety.[13]

Another unique consideration when working with children and adults with a communication disability is the acoustic and lighting environment in which clinical interactions occur. It is well known that the presence of noise, reverberation, and visual distractions can impact one's ability to communicate. While these effects can be more pronounced for people with a hearing loss, even people with typical hearing can experience difficulties communicating in noisy, distracting environments. Poor acoustics not only makes it challenging for individuals to hear one another, it can also increase the effort required to communicate. Optimal acoustic environments can improve not only speech intelligibility between communication partners, but there is also evidence that clinicians experience less pressure, are less irritable, and are more relaxed when working in an improved acoustic environment.[14] In a similar vein, ample natural lighting can have communication benefits for patients and family members, along with a range of psychosocial benefits.[2,3,12]

Importantly, the consideration of the physical environment does not have to be restricted to the clinical consultation room; the same principles apply to the entire organizational setting. For example, most clinical settings have patient waiting rooms, and this space should not be forgotten as an opportunity for promoting PFCC. The inclusion of toys and play opportunities within the waiting room has been found to relieve anxiety in children, as has aromatherapy for adults.[13] Another element which may not be appropriate for the consultation room, but has merit in the waiting room, is the presence of soft background music which has been shown to reduce patient stress and anxiety.[12,13]

Student Activity 3.2: Consideration of the Listening Environment

The acoustics of a room, and therefore the quality of a room's listening environment, can be impacted by room design and furnishings. Before referring to ▶ Fig. 3.3, think about ways in which you think room design and furnishings may help or hinder the acoustics of a typical clinic room. Brainstorm ways in which clinicians could improve the acoustics of their clinic spaces.

Room acoustic and lighting problems	Possible solutions
Noise from heating, ventilation, and air conditioning systems	• Close doors and windows, remembering that even a small opening can let in a considerable amount of noise • Provide sound-absorbing surfaces (e.g., sound absorbing panels, curtains)
High ceilings	• Install carpet or rugs on the floor • Attach rubber seals or plastic foam strips to reduce the leakage of sounds through windows and doors
Noise from tables, chairs, and pedestrian traffic	• Cover hard surfaces with cloth, cushions • Arrange furniture so that the person with a communication disability does not have to face any strong light
Noise from medical equipment	• Adapt window coverings to minimize glare • Be mindful of the impact of shiny surfaces on glare • Use soft room lighting

Fig. 3.3 The impact of décor and design on room acoustics and lighting and possible solutions to improve the listening environment.

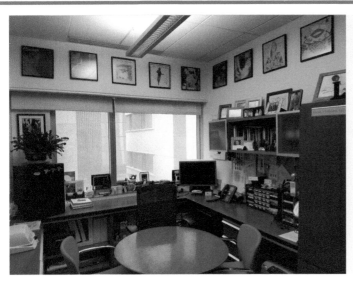

Fig. 3.4 A patient- and family-centered clinical space demonstrating the placement of personal effects.

3.2.4 Personal Effects

When you viewed **Videos 3.1** and **3.2**, you might have also noticed the addition of personal effects within the rooms by way of personal photographs and belongings of the clinician. Why would this be an important feature of a patient- and family-centered clinical space? One of the key components of PFCC is the development of an effective relationship between the patient, family, and clinician. In order to develop trusting professional relationships, clinicians sometimes choose to disclose personal information about themselves. Although the degree of self-disclosure may vary depending on the patient, his or her family, and the clinician's personal preference, some level of self-disclosure is often beneficial. In the physical clinical environment, this self-disclosure may take one of many forms, but will generally reflect who the clinician is as a person (e.g., personal photographs, travel memorabilia, thank you cards, and personalized calendars). As an example, Joseph Montano, an audiologist in New York, has taken a moment to share his clinical space (▶ Fig. 3.4) and his reflections on how to create an environment of care (see the box on next page "A Word from a Clinical Expert: Creating an Environment of Care").

3.3 Products and Technology

Within the ICF, there is an entire chapter dedicated to the important role that products and technology play in the environment for people with a disability and their family members. Essentially, in order to address the three main facets of PFCC (i.e., effective therapeutic relationship between the patient,

family, and clinician; patient- and family-driven care; and incorporation of patient and family needs, preferences, and biopsychosocial context), optimal communication and education is vital. This may take the form of more general products and technology within the clinic space which are readily available to you, as the clinician, your patients, and their family members; or these products and technology may be specifically adapted or designed for you, your patients, or their families (▶ Fig. 3.2).

Indeed, it is not just the World Health Organization that highlights the importance of products and technology for providing access to optimal communication for people with communication disability. One guiding principle of the United Nation's Convention on the Rights of Persons with Disabilities stipulates in Article 9 that in order to enable persons with disabilities to live independently and participate in daily activities, all appropriate measures should be taken to provide access "to information and communications, including information and communication technologies and systems."[15] What does this mean for speech–language pathologists and audiologists working with people with communication disability? Simply, this means that clinicians have a responsibility to do all that is possible to provide accessible options for communication, including the use of general and specific products and technology.

3.3.1 Products and Technology for Communication

It is important that a range of communication methods are used during all stages of the clinical

Joseph Montano, Audiologist, United States

Just for a moment, I'm going to take you back to Lorna who you met in Chapter 1. Lorna could be considered a typical patient deciding to seek a consultation with an audiologist for the first time. She is an older adult, and if she possesses the characteristics of the average hearing health seeking individual, then it would be expected that she has a moderate sensorineural hearing loss, and may be somewhat apprehensive about the entire process. She has been thinking about this for a long time, perhaps 10 years or so, but hasn't been able to prioritize it because of her caring responsibilities for Shane. Now that she has amassed the courage to make the necessary appointments, she is faced with a series of decisions which she may not want to make nor feel capable of making. In order to ease Lorna into the hearing health care arena, it is our responsibility to create the environment of care, one that is conducive to PFCC.

ASHA refers to audiologic rehabilitation as an ecological process that encompasses all aspects of the environment of a patient with hearing loss.[16] That would include, not only the communication environments that patients live in on a daily basis, but the environments that clinicians create when providing rehabilitation. In order for a biopsychosocial treatment model to be effective, a treatment atmosphere must be created that will enable an open communication exchange between the patient, family, and clinician. In order to achieve this, many of the obstacles created by the medical model of service delivery must be overcome. Each audiologist must create a practice environment within the confines of his or her office setting, for example, even a practice located in a hospital-based setting can be modified to allow for PFCC. Regardless of the physical location, creating the appropriate atmosphere is a matter of both behavior and décor. ▶ Fig. 3.4 shows an office practice established within a hospital-based environment. Note that while the setting surrounding the office may seem "medical," the practice location is more conducive to communication. The room is decorated with framed music album covers and there is a relaxed comfortable feeling reflected in the setup. This is a major change from the sterile medical examination rooms most patients are familiar with and helps ease conversation and ensuing discussions.

Creating a Family-Centered Office

Establishing a comfortable environment of care requires buy-in from the entire staff. This would include appointment, clerical and billing staff. Even before the patient meets the clinician, there should be a welcoming atmosphere created during the initial interactions. Scheduling the appointment is particularly important. If possible, the appointment time should be scheduled when it is possible for the patient to attend with a family member. Family involvement should be encouraged from the onset of the inquiry. When they arrive, signage should be clear and easy to follow particularly in locations within large urban health care centers. The waiting room should be comfortable with reading materials available. Communication education materials can be available, but it is not recommended that the waiting room be used for marketing any therapeutic devices.

The Greeting

The typical medical model experience is that a patient is greeted by the receptionist, given a stack of forms to complete, eventually brought into an examination room, and made to wait until the clinician is ready. This model, however, reduces the importance of the initial greeting, a crucial component of the counseling process and relationship development (Montano[17]). As an audiologist in an urban academic medical environment, I am located in the heart of the medical model. Although it may seem obvious and common practice to some, I always go directly to the waiting room and greet my patients and their families. That small effort has a great impact on the development of our clinical relationship. It sets up the equality of the patient, family, and clinician and is the opening for future communication experiences. It creates that horizontal practice plane highly valued in the biopsychosocial method of service delivery. As a result of this practice, numerous positive comments have been made in patient satisfaction surveys about the initial greeting, with patients and families being pleased that their clinician took the time to come and greet them and accompany them into the consultation room. Do not underestimate the importance of a welcoming presence.

Continued ▶

Another historic symbol of the medical model is the white lab coat. A practitioner wearing a white coat immediately sets up an artificial barrier to relationship building. It implies, "I am the doctor; you are the patient." It is a symbol of the top down medical model and an obstacle to an effective therapeutic relationship. While it is necessary sometimes to wear protective clothing when clinicians might be exposed to blood or bodily fluids, white coats are neither necessary nor recommended for counseling patients and families about communication disability.

Setting Up the Room

Technology is a vital part of how we practice as speech–language pathologists and audiologists. The room in which we meet and counsel our patients is important with the technology taking a back seat to the interpersonal relationship. Patients continue to complain that health care providers spend too much time looking at the computer screen. This is particularly problematic when a patient has a hearing loss and requires visual cues for communication. Setting up the room for PFCC should attempt to create an inviting environment that welcomes the participation of both the patient and the family. Seating should be arranged so that all participants have good access to visual cues and are obviously part of the conversation. The clinician sitting behind an office desk with two chairs across from him or her does not create an atmosphere for an equal exchange of communication. In contrast, this type of room design sets up a hierarchy with the clinician clearly in charge. In order to create an interactive environment, the use of a round table as an office centerpiece will invite and encourage all parties to participate. So put down the paper and pencil, move away from the computer, and engage the patient and family in conversation. Learn the patient's story and develop a plan that is workable together as a unit for rehabilitation.

process, including referral, confirmation of appointment, assessment and intervention, and follow-up. These forms of communication may include information and communication technologies, as well as assistive products and technology.

Information and communication technologies include all technologies that allow for an exchange of information, such as optical and auditory devices (e.g., headphones, reading glasses), audio recorders and receivers, videoconferencing equipment, telephone devices, internet, and e-mail. To communicate with patients and families in a patient- and family-centered manner, it is important that clinicians identify patient and family member preferences regarding mode of communication and be flexible with the way in which information is sent and received.

Importantly, to be patient- and family-centered, clinicians must also be aware of the need to use specialized assistive products and technology when communicating with some patients and family members. This is especially important in speech–language pathology and audiology where the very nature of the patient's communication disability implies that communication may need to be supported or enhanced through the use of specialized assistive products and technology. Family members may also have specific communication needs which clinicians should be aware of, and indeed it might be the case that you, as the clinician, will have your own communication device needs. Assistive products and technology for communication that patients, family members, and yourself may use include prescription glasses and contact lenses; cochlear implants, hearing aids, and/or FM systems; voice prostheses; and augmentative and AAC systems (e.g., communication boards and speech-generating devices). However, merely having the products and technology available will not necessarily assist communication, and therefore it is important that the patient, family, and clinician use them appropriately to ensure that communication within the clinical environment is optimal. Alison Moorcroft, a speech–language pathologist, describes how the use of AAC can promote PFCC, and how speech–language pathologists and audiologists can facilitate the use of AAC systems with patients and family members who use them (see box on next page "A Word from a Clinical Expert: Barriers and Facilitators to AAC Use").

A Word from a Clinical Expert: Barriers and Facilitators to AAC Use

Alison Moorcroft, Speech–Language Pathologist, Australia

The appropriate use of communication systems are of utmost importance, as patients and families have reported inadequate health care experiences when clinicians do not know how to use systems,[18] do not make time to use systems with the patients,[19] or believe that using systems is not a part of their role.[20] Understandably, such experiences do not fit the desired model of PFCC, and can result in a variety of physical and psychosocial consequences. For example, adults with complex communication needs report that communication barriers in the hospital environment mean they are unable to participate in their own diagnoses and health management[18] and therefore lack control over what happens to them.[21] In some instances, they may feel frustrated, angry, depressed, and unsafe, and researchers have associated a lack of communication success in hospital with an increased length of stay.[18] AAC users and their families acknowledge that communication is difficult at times, however, expect clinicians to at least "have a go" and attempt communication despite the potential for errors.[19]

Communication with patients with complex communication needs can be facilitated by observing how family members use the system,[22] asking them for help when communication breaks down, following written directives for communication provided by the patient or his or her family, and asking the patient, family members, or another professional how to make communication with the patient more effective.[23] It is of equal importance to then share this information with other health professionals and in that way support the patients to ensure that they are consistently provided with the optimal environment for communication.[23] Together, these strategies will best enable the patient to be an active participant in his or her speech–language pathology and audiology management.

Despite the documented benefits of AAC systems for people with complex communication needs, AAC users and their families may neglect to bring the system to all environments,[21,24,25] or have a system that does not meet the language demands of the current environment.[19] In such circumstances, clinicians can remain patient- and family-centered by having generic AAC systems prepared and available, and making basic communication boards for a specific need.[22] Parents have also suggested providing written information in symbol form to further promote the patient as an active participant in their care.[19] This modification is in line with broader discussions around the importance of accessible health care information (e.g., aphasia-friendly documentation) as discussed later in this chapter. However, it is important to acknowledge that some patients will not accept or utilize the assistive products and technology made available to them. This resistance spans a variety of products, including AAC systems,[26,27] hearing aids, and other assistive technology.[28] In such circumstances, it is important to acknowledge the patients as the primary drivers of their health care, and respect their autonomy by communicating with them in their preferred manner.

So how do you get products and technology in the environment ready for PFCC? On next page is a checklist that can be used to ensure you have the products and technology available for optimal communication (▶ Fig. 3.5). By way of example, we have completed the checklist as the speech–language pathologist working with Miranda, Flynn, and their son Andrew in our early intervention program (▶ Fig. 3.6).

3.3.2 General Products and Technology for Education

In addition to ensuring that you make optimal use of products and technology for communicating with patients and family members, the way in which you provide education is also an important consideration for being a patient- and family-centered clinician. Education can be provided

Clinician	Communication preferences
	Glasses/ contact lenses
	Hearing aids/ cochlear implants
	FM system
	Communication board
	Voice prosthesis
	Other
	Other
Patient	Communication preferences
	Glasses/ contact lenses
	Hearing aids/ cochlear implants
	FM system
	Communication board
	Voice prosthesis
	Other
	Other
Family members	Communication preferences
	Glasses/ contact lenses
	Hearing aids/ cochlear implants
	FM system
	Communication board
	Voice prosthesis
	Other
	Other

Fig. 3.5 Checklist to help ensure that you have the products and technology available for optimal communication between you, your patients, and their family members.

using a number of different products, in a number of different modes, with the purpose of imparting knowledge, expertise, or skills (▶ Fig. 3.2). For example, clinicians can educate patients and their family members through books, manuals, fact sheets, information brochures, DVDs, websites, podcasts, and educational toys. These educational resources can be available for patients and their family members in your waiting room, clinic room, and/or for personal use at home.

Educational books can take many forms, for example, they could be a simple textbook written about the patient's health condition, memoirs written by patients and their family members, and specific workbooks designed to complement therapeutic programs. Manuals should accompany devices that patients and their family members might be using, such as hearing aids and AAC devices. Fact sheets and information brochures can be used to provide patients and their family members with both general and specific information about their communication disability or the treatment program.

Importantly, however, in order to be a patient- and family-centered clinician, this education must be provided to patients and family in a range of different formats and modalities, including in hardcopy and electronic formats, and it must be provided in an accessible format. For this information to be accessible, it is important that it adheres to universal best practice guidelines for written health information. This is especially important given that approximately one-third of adults in the United States have basic or below basic health

Clinician	Communication preferences	
	Glasses/ contact lenses ✓	
	Hearing aids/ cochlear implants	
	FM system	
	Communication board	
	Voice prosthesis	
	Other	
	Other	
Patient	Communication preferences *verbal ; keyword sign* ✓	
	Glasses/ contact lenses	
	Hearing aids/ cochlear implants	
	FM system	
	Communication board	
	Voice prosthesis	
	Other *Communication book* ✓	
	Other *Social stories* ✓	
Family members	Communication preferences	
	Glasses/ contact lenses *Miranda — glasses; Flynn — contacts* ✓	
	Hearing aids/ cochlear implants	
	FM system	
	Communication board	
	Voice prosthesis	
	Other	
	Other	

Fig. 3.6 Sample checklist to help ensure that you have the products and technology available for optimal communication between you, Andrew, Flynn, and Miranda.

literacy.[29] Health literacy is defined as the ability to "access, understand, appraise, and apply health information in order to make judgments and take decisions in everyday life concerning health care, disease prevention, and health promotion to maintain or improve quality of life…."[30] (p.3). A systematic review, which looked at the impact of health literacy on health outcomes, revealed that low health literacy was associated with poorer health-related knowledge and poorer health status.[31]

First and foremost, clinicians should be aware of the readability of any information they provide to patients and their family members, including not only educational information but also written assessment reports and letters. It is generally recommended that written health information have a reading grade level lower than 6, meaning that someone with 6 years of formal education should be able to understand what is written.

How do you calculate the readability of written health information that you give your patients and family members, in a Microsoft Word document?

If using a PC, follow these simple steps (applicable to Microsoft™ Word 2016):
1. Click **File** and then click **Options**.
2. Click **Proofing**.
3. Make sure **"show readability statistics"** is selected and press OK.
4. Click **Review** and **Spelling and Grammar**.
5. After the spelling and grammar check is complete, the readability statistics will be displayed. Play close attention to the **Flesch–Kincaid grade level**.

If using a Mac, follow these simple steps:
1. Click **Word** and then click **Preferences**.
2. Click **Spelling and Grammar**.
3. Make sure that **"show readability statistics"** is selected.
4. Click **Tools** and **Spelling and Grammar**.
5. After the spelling and grammar check is complete, the readability statistics will be displayed. Play close attention to the **Flesch–Kincaid grade level**.

Please note: These steps will differ depending on the version of Microsoft Word you are using, as well as the Operating System. If the above steps don't work, search online for what will work for you.

When formatting written health information, try to stick to the following principles:
• Use small amounts of text.
• Use short, simple sentences, highlighting key words.
• Use simple language that is straight to the point.
• Avoid the use of jargon.
• Write in the first or second person.
• Use a minimum 14-point font.
• Use bold text headings and borders to emphasize key points.
• Use distinctive headings that link to the content.
• Try to avoid the use of *italics* and capitalization.
• Avoid the use of judgmental language.
• Avoid abbreviations.
• Include graphics.

A study of hearing aid user guides has found that they are typically poorly designed to help people who wear hearing aids to learn how to use and manage their hearing aids![33] Lorna who was introduced to you in the first chapter of the book has a mild–moderate sensorineural hearing loss and is considering trying hearing aids. ▶ Fig. 3.7 shows an example of information from a typical hearing aid user guide that Lorna might receive and ▶ Fig. 3.8 shows an example of a best practice hearing aid user guide developed based on the Helpful Tips above. Compare the two figures and make a list of the differences between them. How do you think Lorna might react if she was given the typical hearing aid user guide in ▶ Fig. 3.7?

In addition to the reading grade level, you will need to take into consideration the formatting that is used (e.g., font size and type, white space, use of pictures/diagrams); the language complexity of text (sentence length; jargon; complex, multisyllabic words); and the type of information provided, such as placing emphasis on the "how to" information.[32] As an aside, clinicians should also be mindful of their verbal communication when providing education to patients and their families and ensure they are not using clinical jargon unnecessarily. For other "top tips," for ensuring the information you provide patients and their families is easily accessible, refer to a short article developed by the National Center for Health Marketing, Centers for Disease Control and Prevention: https://www.cdc.gov/healthcommunication/pdf/healthliteracy.pdf

3.3.3 Assistive Products and Technology for Education

Above, we highlighted that the health literacy of patients and their families needs to be taken into consideration when providing products and technology for education purposes. Importantly, there are times when products and technology should

Direct Audio Input (DAI)

Using the Direct Audio Input socket enables direct, undisturbed connection to facilities such as: Television · Radio · Remote microphone.

How to connect the audio boot to the hearing instrument: Pay close attention to the illustrations on how to connect and disconnect the audio boot below.
1. Make sure the tip of the audio boot is placed firstly in the HIAI (Hearing Instrument Accessories Interface).
2. Click the audio boot on to the hearing instrument.
3. The audio boot is now connected.

Low Battery Warning

Your hearing care professional can activate a Low Battery Warning function in your hearing instruments. When the battery voltage/power decreases to a certain level, the instrument will emit five soft "beeping" signals. This sequence will continue every five minutes until the instrument automatically switches off. The occurrence of the sequence can differ by using rechargeable batteries and also between different battery brands. It is recommended that you keep a spare battery on hand.

Changing the Battery

1. Gently push the battery compartment to open.
2. Use a magnet pin to remove the battery, if at hand.
3. After removing the old battery, insert the new one. It is important to insert the battery with the positive side in the correct position. The battery door has a + marking to help determine correct insertion.
4. Always use Zinc-Air or rechargeable batteries size 312 (61 model) and #13 for (71& 81 models)

Tip

Removing the battery when you are not wearing the instrument for a longer period will help prevent corrosion of the battery contacts.

9

Maintenance

Daily Maintenance

It is important to keep your hearing instrument clean and dry every day. To clean the instrument, use a soft cloth. If the instrument has been exposed to high humidity or perspiration, use a drying kit that is available from your hearing care professional.

To avoid the need for repairs:
1. Never immerse the instrument in water or other liquids since this may cause permanent damage to the hearing instrument.
2. Protect your hearing instrument from rough handling, and avoid dropping it on hard surfaces or floors.
3. Do not leave the instrument in or near direct heat or sunlight since excessive heat can damage the instrument or deform the casing.

Cleaning the Earmould

The earmould should be cleaned regularly:
1. Remove the earmould and the tubing from the hearing instrument before you clean it.
2. To clean the earmould, rinse with lukewarm water.
3. If ear wax is stuck in the sound canal of the earmould, the cleaning loop or a syringe with lukewarm water can be used to "push" the wax out.
4. Blow gently through the tubing to remove moisture trapped inside.
5. Be sure to thoroughly dry the earmould and its tubing before reconnecting it to the hearing instrument.

The tubing connecting the earmould to the hearing instrument should be changed if it becomes stiff or brittle. Contact your hearing care professional to change the tubing when needed.

10

Fig. 3.7 Pages from a typical hearing aid user guide.

be further adapted or specifically designed for individual patients and their family members. This is particularly relevant for speech–language pathologists and audiologists given that we are working with patients who have a communication disability.

Although there may be a number of different patients and family members for which speech–language pathologists and audiologists need to specifically design information, one very relevant example is information provided to patients with aphasia. Best practice guidelines for the management of people with aphasia are summarized at http://www.aphasiapathway.com.au/ and they emphasize the need to create accessible communication environments. A component of that is providing written educational materials at numerous points that meet the preferences and needs of people with aphasia

and their families throughout the patient's journey (i.e., immediately poststroke as well as in the medium and long term). This is particularly challenging because of the reading language deficits that are a part of the communication disability experienced by people with aphasia. There is a body of literature that has described the components and benefits of "aphasia-friendly" written materials for patients with aphasia. For example, Rose et al.[34] investigated the design preferences of 40 adults with aphasia and found that, on average, they preferred the following:
• Numbers to be expressed as figures rather than words.
• 14-point font.
• Verdana font style.
• 1.5 line spacing.
• The inclusion of graphics, preferably photographs.

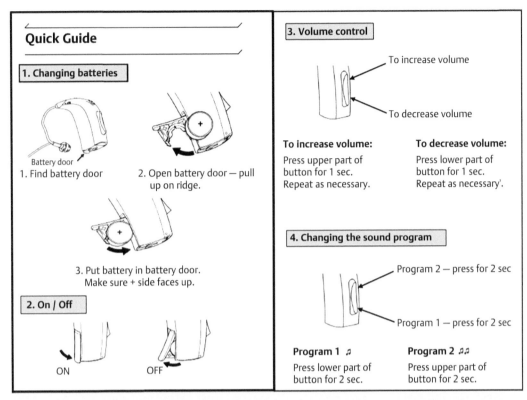

Quick Guide

1. Changing batteries

Battery door
1. Find battery door

2. Open battery door — pull up on ridge.

3. Put battery in battery door. Make sure + side faces up.

2. On / Off

ON   OFF

3. Volume control

To increase volume

To decrease volume

To increase volume:
Press upper part of button for 1 sec. Repeat as necessary.

To decrease volume:
Press lower part of button for 1 sec. Repeat as necessary'.

4. Changing the sound program

Program 2 — press for 2 sec

Program 1 — press for 2 sec

Program 1 ♪
Press lower part of button for 2 sec.

Program 2 ♪♪
Press upper part of button for 2 sec.

Fig. 3.8 Pages from a best practice hearing aid user guide.

Interesting Fact

What do people with aphasia think about the written health information they have been given by health professionals?

People with aphasia typically find information too complex to understand, which can be very distressing. Below is a quote from a patient with aphasia. To learn more about the experiences of patients with aphasia accessing written health information, we direct you to the original publication.[35]

"Oh re ridiculous...Well ah you think you're a ...university student before you can understand them...it's just beyond. Throw it away because I can't understand...too complicated!" (p. 373)[35] (person with aphasia referring to reading a health information brochure).

3.4 Support, Relationships, and Attitudes

Until this point, the focus has been on preparing the physical environment to be patient- and family-centered. Importantly, however, in order to practice PFCC, the people in the environment are a key consideration. The ICF provides a comprehensive coding system to represent the support, relationships, and attitudes of a range of people in a patient's environment.[1] The ICF recognizes that these people could include immediate and extended family, friends, acquaintances, neighbors, health professionals, and other professionals (▶ Fig. 3.9). As a patient- and family-centered clinician, you must consider and subsequently address the amount of physical and emotional support, nurturing, protection, and assistance provided to patients and their families by these people, including people in their home, workplace, and other daily activities. Similarly, patient- and family-centered clinicians must consider the general or specific attitudes, opinions, and beliefs the aforementioned people have that may influence your patients' and their family members' individual behaviors or actions.[1]

Given the diverse and complicated nature of relationships and social networks, it can sometimes be helpful to use social network analysis to identify the key people in a patient's life (▶ Fig. 3.10).[36] As part of this activity, patients are asked to name people who are most important to them, and typically, the people who they communicate most often with, in the inner circle. Next, patients are asked to name people who are still important, but not as much as those in the inner circle, in the second ring. Finally, patients are asked to identify people in their network who they interact with on a regular basis, but who are less important; their names are written in the outer ring. Given that the attitudes and support provided by all people within a patient's social network are likely to influence patient outcomes, you need to be cognizant of the attitudes they might hold and work to maximize the strengths that the network members might bring to the patient. It will also be important to identify any network members who are particularly challenging for your patient and identify the support that the patient and the family need to address the challenges. For example, many patients with hearing impairment describe the difficulties they face when communicating with specific individuals in their social network: "My grandchildren are so hard to hear—they speak softly and never look at me" is a common patient complaint.

Code	Definition
e310 Immediate family and **e315 Extended family**	Individuals related by birth, family, marriage or other relationship recognized by the culture as immediate or extended family.
e320 Friends	Individuals who are close and ongoing participants in relationships characterized by trust and mutual support.
e325 Acquaintances, peers, colleagues, neighbours and community members	Individuals who are familiar to each other as acquaintances, peers, colleagues, neighbours, and community members, in situations of work, school, recreation, or other aspect of life, and who share demographic features such as age, gender, religious creed or ethnicity or pursue common interests.
e355 Health professionals	All service providers working within the context of the health system, such as doctors, nurses, physiotherapists, occupational therapists, speech therapists, audiologists, and medical social workers.
e360 Other professional	All service providers working outside the health system, including social workers, lawyers, teachers, architects, and designers.

Fig. 3.9 Relevant environmental factors related to support, relationships, and attitudes for patient- and family-centered speech pathology and audiology.

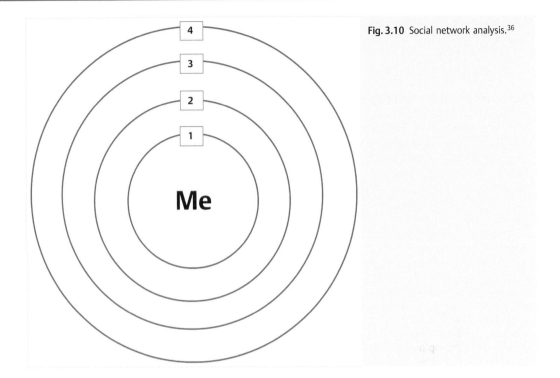

Fig. 3.10 Social network analysis.[36]

Using the social network analysis tool shown in ▶ Fig. 3.10, we would like you to think about Miranda and Flynn, and brainstorm who in their social network may be providing support for them as they care for their son Andrew.

Now contrast this social network with the likely network of Emily, who you also met in Chapter 1 by completing the social network analysis tool for her. As a young adult, Emily is likely to have a different social network than that of a couple with a young child. Perhaps her network would be more like yours as a student speech–language pathologist or audiologist.

In the same way that family member attitudes can impact the care of a patient with a communication disability, so can your own attitude as the speech–language pathologist or audiologist working with the patient. It is being increasingly documented in the literature that speech–language pathologists and audiologists believe in and have a preference for delivering PFCC.[37–42] Interestingly, the clinician's workplace setting has been found to play a role in speech–language pathologists and audiologists preferences for PFCC, with speech–language pathologists working in private practice showing stronger preferences for PFCC compared to speech–language pathologists working in educational settings[41]; and audiologists working in community education, industry, and teaching having greater preferences for PFCC than audiologists working in private practice and adult assessment.[38] Similarly, a clinician's age and years of work experience can also influence these attitudes toward PFCC.[38] The Institute for Patient- and Family-Centered Care has published a checklist for health professionals so you can reflect on your own attitude about working with patients and families. It can be used individually or as a tool to generate discussion between colleagues about PFCC. Click on the link to access this checklist: http://www.ipfcc.org/resources/Checklist_for_Attitudes.pdf

Despite many individual clinicians having a positive attitude toward PFCC, gaps have been identified between beliefs and actual implementation, with research indicating that a number of principles of PFCC are not consistently incorporated into their everyday work with patients and families.[37, 41,43–49] This may suggest that the positive attitude of the individual clinician may not be sufficient for the implementation of PFCC, rather, there are other professionals and broader services, systems, and policies that might be the mediating factors to implementation. Below, Rebecca Bennett, an audiologist, describes how clinicians, managers, administrative staff, and the service as a whole can provide support for a PFCC approach.

A Word from a Research and Clinical Expert: A Whole Team Approach to Applying PFCC in an Organization

Rebecca Bennett, Audiologist, Australia

A PFCC approach to health care does not only reside on the interaction between the patient, family, and clinician, but also managers and administration staff who are responsible for ensuring patients and their families receive optimal care throughout the entire health care experience. PFCC strategies can be adopted and supported at all levels of the organization. For example:

Clinicians should ...

- Make a conscious effort to engage family members in appointments.
- Change their language.
- Change their clinical processes, such as use of shared decision making tools, educational booklets, group education sessions.
- Prompt themselves to change old habits.

Managers should ...

- Create and support a PFCC workplace by emphasizing the value and importance of PFCC in all correspondence with staff.
- Lead changes in administrative and clinical protocols to incorporate PFCC approaches to care.
- Train, engage, and support staff in PFCC practices, including communication and empathy skills.
- Allow time for planning, training, and implementation of PFCC protocols and practices.

Administrative staff should ...

- Encourage patients to bring family members to appointments by describing the benefits of their involvement.
- Collect information about patient and family preferences for care.
- Elicit and support patient and family choices, including preferred appointment days/times, location of consultation, and preferred clinician.
- Respond to patient and family queries in a timely manner.
- Use simple and friendly language and provide clear and easy-to-understand information.
- Interact with patients in the waiting room, ensuring patient comfort.
- Maintain a tidy and inviting waiting room space.
- Understand and respect patients' and families' rights to access their own medical information and provide willingly when requested.

Health services, systems, and policies should ...

- Pay attention to the physical environment by creating calm and welcoming spaces; providing consultation rooms with sufficient space and additional chairs for families to be involved; ensuring that health services have parking spaces and/or public transport nearby; and providing parent facilities and change rooms.
- Provide easy access to care by having simple appointment making processes (e.g., online bookings); minimizing wait times for appointments and treatments; having payment options, such as payment plans and access to government rebates; providing a range of service delivery options (e.g., offsite or home appointments); and putting in place clear referral pathways.
- Take advantage of available information technologies, such as online self-management tools or apps and patient management systems that capture patient preferences.
- Prioritize communication processes, including clear signage to and within the building; including maps, directions, and transport and parking options in appointment reminder letters; and billing statements itemized in clear language.

Given the importance of all staff working within an organization having a shared understanding of PFCC, including administrative staff, break into pairs and role play the below two scenarios. One of you should play the role of the patient and one of you should play the role of the staff member, and then swap for the second scenario. Think carefully about how the administrative staff member or the audiologist could respond to the patient in a patient- and family-centered way:

1. An administrative staff member receives a phone call from a patient to say that his wife is complaining that her hearing has gotten worse, that she had her hearing tested 3 years ago, at which point they purchased hearing aids, but that she never used the hearing aids and believes they were a waste of money.
2. Repeat the scenario, but this time instead of the patient telling his story to the administrative staff members, he tells it to the audiologist at the beginning of the clinical consultation.

3.5 Health Services, Systems, and Policies

Given the crucial role that services, systems, and policies play in supporting organizational change toward being more patient- and family-centered, we deem it important to now turn to issues about implementation of PFCC within an organization, and what role you could play as a speech–language pathologist or audiologist. Rebecca Bennett, an audiologist with experience in implementing a patient- and family-centered audiologic service in Australia, shared some of her insights (see box on right column "A Word from a Research and Clinical Expert: Creating a Culture of PFCC in the Workplace").

You can also view **Video 3.4** to hear how Bettina Turnball has managed the implementation of PFCC in her organisation.

Rebecca Bennett, Audiologist, Australia
In the same way that PFCC is about seeing the patient and his or her family as a unit with individual needs and unique experiences of their health condition, organizations implementing PFCC strategies must also recognize their staff as individuals with unique experiences that may help or hinder the implementation process. Reducing staff resistance to the implementation of PFCC can be assisted by ensuring that staff understand the reasons behind the change, agree that change is needed, and are actively engaged in the process of implementing PFCC practices. Although PFCC programs are most successful when implemented from the top, staff within the organization can still play a pivotal role in ensuring PFCC practices are successfully adopted. Damschroder et al[50] identifies three types of leaders within an organization: (1) formally appointed leaders, such as team leaders or middle managers; (2) opinion leaders, who are individuals within the organization who have formal or informal influence on the attitudes and beliefs of their colleagues; and (3) champions, who dedicate themselves to supporting, marketing, and overcoming resistance to change within the organization. Students or staff wanting to support PFCC practices in the workplace could become champions in working toward and building a PFCC culture in the workplace.

When implementing a PFCC strategy in a workplace, the organization needs the following:
- Strong committed senior leadership.
- A strategic vision of PFCC clearly and constantly communicated to internal and external stakeholders.
- Involvement of patients and families in the development of the strategy.
- A supportive work environment for all employees.
- Regular measurement and feedback of PFCC.
- Adequate resourcing for health care delivery design.
- To build staff capacity to support PFCC.
- Accountability and incentives for the provision of PFCC.
- Supportive information technology for the delivery of PFCC.
- A culture strongly supportive of change and learning.

Dr Michelle Bennett, Speech–Language Pathologist, Australia

The training and practice of allied health professionals has undergone a significant shift over the past two decades. Traditional medical models of service delivery have made way for care that is less directed by the health professional and is more inclusive of the individual needs, preferences, and contribution of the patient. The principles of PFCC underlie the core values taught within many allied health professions today, and the relatively "new" model of care introduced to Australia, "consumer-directed" care (CDC).

Requiring a strong foundation of PFCC but shifting care even further along the continuum, CDC aims to provide the person receiving the health service (the "consumer") with increased choice and control over his or her health care. In CDC, the health professional must be open to explore new or additional services as "directed" by the consumer. The health professional is still ethically obliged to provide the consumer with sufficient information to make an informed decision about his or her health care needs and to provide evidenced-based health care; however, the decision of what services are received, what goals are set, and how services are funded ultimately resides with the consumer. The intended outcome of CDC, for the consumer, is the ability to exercise greater choice and control over his or her own health outcomes and health care.

Several potential ethical issues surrounding CDC have been raised. How will patients and their families be supported in making informed decisions about their care needs? Can consumers be expected to know how to seek government-provided funds and how to allocate funds to meet their short- and long-term needs? Can we expect a consumer to be able to determine whether a service provided to him or her is evidenced-based and the most effective means of meeting his or her needs? With the introduction of CDC in Australia in its infancy we do not yet have clear answers to these questions. As a clinician then, how do we support our patients and their families, our "consumers" to participate in CDC? How do we ensure that within our chosen profession we continue to adhere to our obligation to provide ethical and evidence-based health care while also fostering consumer choice, and flexibility and innovation in the services we provide?

As speech–language pathologists and audiologists we know that many of our patients will have physical, sensory, cognitive, and/or communication difficulties that limit their ability to participate in CDC unless appropriate supports are in place to assist their participation. We know that many of our patients will have difficulty understanding their health care needs, the service options available to them, and the funding systems available to support their care. We also know that many of our patients will have difficulty expressing their needs and preferences, and advocating for their choices. So where do we start? The first step in supporting our patients with CDC is to ensure we understand the intention of CDC and how CDC is being implemented in the service in which we are working. As a model of care focused on choice and flexibility, in practice, CDC will look a little different across individual health services and individual consumers. There is no "recipe" for CDC. We must do as we always have—evaluate our patients' and families' needs and capabilities and determine what strategies will best assist them to achieve their health care goals, including goals surrounding their involvement in care planning and decision making. We must remember that our role is not only treating the communication disability, but also as a consultant and advocate for our patients and families.

A service equipped to provide CDC will already be delivering services consistent with PFCC, with patients and families featured at the center of all care decisions and service planning. The service will, however, have the intent and resources needed to take this focus a step further. For staff to embrace CDC, a management structure and approach that fosters both flexibility and innovation is essential, as is the provision of appropriate professional development to support staff in working flexibly and embracing new innovations. The consumer must also be informed about the intent of CDC, how CDC is being implemented in the service, and the important role of the consumer in CDC. For some older patients and families, taking a more active role in their health care may not be a role they are initially comfortable with or wish to take. Importantly though, their choice to be "more" or "less" involved in their care planning is an integral part of CDC that needs to be respected and supported. If you are working within an organization that provides CDC, the checklist provided in ▶ Fig. 3.11 may be helpful in checking the level of understanding and support for this approach from the perspective of the service, staff, and consumers.

The service I am working in:		
1. Has a clear mission statement and implementation guidelines outlining the commitment of the service to CDC and how the service is implementing CDC?	Yes	No
2. Presents all policy and procedure documents to consumers in an easy English format?	Yes	No
3. Develops service policies and procedures in consultation with consumers and openly invites consumers to regularly review service policies and procedures?	Yes	No
4. Has a clearly defined procedure to ensure all reasonable actions suggested through consumer feedback are carried out by the service?	Yes	No
Staff within the service:		
5. Have a good understanding of the intent of CDC and their role in CDC, and how CDC is being implemented in the service in which they are employed and/or contracted to?	Yes	No
6. Are supported by all levels of management and by their peers to work flexibly and embrace innovation and change in their role and in the roles of others?	Yes	No
7. Are provided with appropriate professional development opportunities to support service innovations and the changing needs and preferences of consumers?	Yes	No
Consumers of the service:		
8. Have a good understanding of the intent of and their role in CDC, and how CDC is being implemented within the service they are engaged with?	Yes	No
9. Are considered by the service, and express themselves as, partners in the delivery of the health service rather than as receivers of care?	Yes	No
10. Are provided with the supports they need to take an active role in their care planning?	Yes	No

Fig. 3.11 Ten-point checklist of consumer-directed care.

In some sectors where speech–language pathologists and audiologists work, there has already been a significant shift toward PFCC. Importantly, these shifts have sometimes been led by Government, and therefore the motivation, support, and attitudes for such change may be different compared to organizations that have independently promoted the shift toward PFCC. Nevertheless, as a patient- and family-centered clinician, you need to be mindful of the impact of this change on your patients and families and how this might influence your overall management.

One example of how this has occurred in Australia is through the introduction of "consumer-directed care" (CDC) within the aged care sector. (See the box on previous page "A Word from a Clinical and Research Expert: Extending Patient- and Family-Centered Care to Consumer-Directed Care in Aged Care Environments"). Michelle Bennett, a speech–language pathologist, with clinical and research experience in applying PFCC and CDC in aged care, shares her perceptions of how this environmental context might impact the way you practice as a patient- and family-centered clinician.

We've reached the end of Chapter 3, and we hope you understand the extent of getting all aspects of the environment ready for PFCC. While you're on clinical placement or after you have graduated and started working as a patient- and family-centered speech–language pathologist or audiologist, one of the best ways to evaluate the extent of patient- and family-centeredness in your organization is by conducting a "walk-about." The Institute for Patient- and Family-Centered Care has published some instructions on how you can obtain the perspectives of patients and their families about all aspects of the environment, including the physical environment, the use of products and technology, the support, relationships and attitudes of staff, and broader systems and policies. The instructions are available here: http://www.ipfcc.org/resources/How_To_Conduct_A_Walk-About.pdf

3.6 Summary

In summary, this chapter has shed light on the full scope of the environment in which people with communication disability and their family members function. We have used the ICF as a framework to understand the breadth of the environment that can influence PFCC. Importantly, this environment not only refers to the physical environment, but also the social and attitudinal environment in which people live and conduct their lives, and the features of the health service, systems, and policies in which you work and patients and families receive care. We have provided practical examples of how you as an individual speech–language pathologist or audiologist can improve the environment for your patients and their families (e.g., embracing communication technology, creating "friendly" accessible written education materials). We have also provided examples of how organizations can improve the environment and highlighted the importance of having buy-in from all levels of the organization for PFCC to occur. We hope that you will become a PFCC champion in your clinical work directly with patients, in your workplace and in your community outside of work.

3.7 Reflections

Please respond to the following reflection questions in your PFCC journal:

1. What are the three environmental factors from the ICF that are relevant to the delivery of PFCC?

2. What are the five examples of assistive technologies that might help patients and families with communication disorders?

3. Consider a recent clinical setting you have worked in as a speech–language pathology or audiology student. How conducive was the physical environment to PFCC? How might it be improved?

References

[1] World Health Organization. ICF, International Classification of Functioning, Disability and Health. Geneva: World Health Organization; 2001

[2] Horowitz S. Optimal healing environments: a prescription for health. Altern Complement Ther. 2008; 14(6):300–305

[3] Ranjbar F, Mahdi Nejad JED. Strategies to design dental clinic for children with mental health promotion approach in the treatment process. Mediterr J Soc Sci. 2016

[4] Scholl I, Zill JM, Härter M, Dirmaier J. An integrative model of patient-centeredness—a systematic review and concept analysis. PLoS One. 2014; 9(9):e107828

[5] Preston P. Proxemics in clinical and administrative settings. J Healthc Manag. 2005; 50(3):151–154

[6] Okken V, van Rompay T, Pruyn A. Exploring space in the consultation room: environmental influences during patient-physician interaction. J Health Commun. 2012; 17(4):397–412

[7] Ajiboye F, Dong F, Moore J, Kallail KJ, Baughman A. Effects of revised consultation room design on patient-physician communication. HERD. 2015; 8(2):8–17

[8] Manav B. Color-emotion associations and color preferences: a case study for residences. Color Res Appl. 2007; 32(2):144–150

[9] Liu W, Ji J, Chen H, Ye C, Androulakis IP. Optimal color design of psychological counseling room by design of experiments and response surface methodology. PLoS One. 2014; 9(3):e90646

[10] Elliot AJ, Maier MA, Moller AC, Friedman R, Meinhardt J. Color and psychological functioning: the effect of red on performance attainment. J Exp Psychol Gen. 2007; 136(1):154–168

[11] Elliot AJ, Maier MA. Color psychology: effects of perceiving color on psychological functioning in humans. Annu Rev Psychol. 2014; 65:95–120

[12] Codinhoto R, Tzortzopoulos P, Kagioglou M, Aouad G, Cooper R. The Impacts of the Built Environment on Health Outcomes. Bradford: Emerald Group Publishing, Limited; 2009:138–151

[13] Biddiss E, Knibbe TJ, McPherson A. The effectiveness of interventions aimed at reducing anxiety in health care waiting spaces: a systematic review of randomized and nonrandomized trials. Anesth Analg. 2014; 119(2):433–448

[14] Blomkvist V, Eriksen CA, Theorell T, Ulrich R, Rasmanis G. Acoustics and psychosocial environment in intensive coronary care. Occup Environ Med. 2005; 62(3):e1

[15] United Nations General Assembly. Convention on the Rights of Persons with Disabilities: Article 9 . https://www.un.org/development/desa/disabilities/convention-on-the-rights-of-persons-with-disabilities/article-9-accessibility.html. Accessed March 15, 2019

[16] American Speech-Language-Hearing Association. Knowledge and skills required for the practice of audiologic/aural rehabilitation [Knowledge and Skills]. www.asha.org/policy. Accessed April 4, 2019

[17] Montano JJ. Overdependence on technology in the management of hearing loss. In R. Goldfarb, (Ed.). Translational Speech-Language Pathology and Audiology. San Diego; Plural Publishing. 2012: 97–105.

[18] Balandin S, Hemsley B, Sigafoos J, Green V. Communicating with nurses: the experiences of 10 adults with cerebral palsy and complex communication needs. Appl Nurs Res. 2007; 20 (2):56–62

[19] Hemsley B, Kuek M, Bastock K, Scarinci N, Davidson B. Parents and children with cerebral palsy discuss communication needs in hospital. Dev Neurorehabil. 2013; 16(6):363–374

[20] Lund SK, Light J. Long-term outcomes for individuals who use augmentative and alternative communication: part III—contributing factors. Augment Altern Commun. 2007; 23(4):323–335

[21] Hemsley B, Balandin S. Without AAC: the stories of unpaid carers of adults with cerebral palsy and complex communication needs in hospital. Augment Altern Commun. 2004; 20 (4):243–258

[22] Hemsley B, Lee S, Munro K, Seedat N, Bastock K, Davidson B. Supporting communication for children with cerebral palsy in hospital: views of community and hospital staff. Dev Neurorehabil. 2014; 17(3):156–166

[23] Finke EH, Light J, Kitko L. A systematic review of the effectiveness of nurse communication with patients with complex communication needs with a focus on the use of augmentative and alternative communication. J Clin Nurs. 2008; 17 (16):2102–2115

[24] Iacono T, Lyon K, Johnson H, West D. Experiences of adults with complex communication needs receiving and using low tech AAC: an Australian context. Disabil Rehabil Assist Technol. 2013; 8(5):392–401

[25] Hemsley B, Balandin S, Worrall L. Nursing the patient with complex communication needs: time as a barrier and a facilitator to successful communication in hospital. J Adv Nurs. 2012; 68(1):116–126

[26] Johnson JM, Inglebret E, Jones C, Ray J. Perspectives of speech language pathologists regarding success versus abandonment of AAC. Augment Altern Commun. 2006; 22(2):85–99

[27] Martin JK, Martin LG, Stumbo NJ, Morrill JH. The impact of consumer involvement on satisfaction with and use of assistive technology. Disabil Rehabil Assist Technol. 2011; 6(3): 225–242

[28] Riemer-Reiss M, Wacker R. Factors associated with assistive technology discontinuance among individuals with disabilities. J Rehabil. 2000; 66(3):44

[29] Kutner M, Greenberg E, Jin Y, Paulsen C. The Health Literacy of America's Adults: Results From the 2003 National Assessment of Adult Literacy (NCES 2006–483). Washington, DC: National Center for Education Statistics; 2006

[30] Sørensen K, Van den Broucke S, Fullam J, et al. (HLS-EU) Consortium Health Literacy Project European. Health literacy and public health: a systematic review and integration of definitions and models. BMC Public Health. 2012; 12(1):80

[31] Dewalt DA, Berkman ND, Sheridan S, Lohr KN, Pignone MP. Literacy and health outcomes: a systematic review of the literature. J Gen Intern Med. 2004; 19(12):1228–1239

[32] Seligman HK, Wallace AS, DeWalt DA, et al. Facilitating behavior change with low-literacy patient education materials. Am J Health Behav. 2007; 31 Suppl 1:S69–S78

[33] Caposecco A, Hickson L, Meyer C. Hearing aid user guides: suitability for older adults. Int J Audiol. 2014; 53 Suppl 1:S43–S51

[34] Rose TA, Worrall LE, Hickson LM, Hoffmann TC. Guiding principles for printed education materials: design preferences of people with aphasia. Int J Speech-Language Pathol. 2012; 14 (1):11–23

[35] Rose TA, Worrall LE, McKenna KT, Hickson LM, Hoffmann TC. Do people with aphasia receive written stroke and aphasia information? Aphasiology. 2009; 23(3):364–392

[36] Kahn RL, Antonucci T. Convoys over the life course: attachment, roles and social support. In: Baltes PB, Brim OG, eds. Life-Span Development and Behavior. New York, NY: Academic Press; 1980:253–286

[37] Crais ER, Roy VP, Free K. Parents' and professionals' perceptions of the implementation of family-centered practices in child assessments. Am J Speech Lang Pathol. 2006; 15(4): 365–377

[38] Laplante-Lévesque A, Hickson L, Grenness C. An Australian survey of audiologists' preferences for patient-centredness. Int J Audiol. 2014; 53 Suppl 1:S76–S82

[39] Manchaiah V, Dockens AL, Bellon-Harn M, Burns ES. Noncongruence between audiologist and patient preferences for patient-centeredness. J Am Acad Audiol. 2017; 28(7):636–643

[40] Manchaiah V, Gomersall PA, Tomé D, Ahmadi T, Krishna R. Audiologists' preferences for patient-centredness: a cross-sectional questionnaire study of cross-cultural differences and similarities among professionals in Portugal, India and Iran. BMJ Open. 2014; 4(10):e005915

[41] Pappas NW, McLeod S, McAllister L, McKinnon DH. Parental involvement in speech intervention: a national survey. Clin Linguist Phon. 2008; 22(4–5):335–344

[42] Meyer C, Scarinci N, Ryan B, Hickson L. "This Is a Partnership Between All of Us": Audiologists' Perceptions of Family Member Involvement in Hearing Rehabilitation. Am J Audiol. 2015; 24(4):536–548

[43] Ali A, Meyer C, Hickson L. Patient-centred hearing care in Malaysia: what do audiologists prefer and to what extent is it implemented in practice? Speech, Language and Hearing. 2017:1–11

[44] Bruce B, Letourneau N, Ritchie J, Larocque S, Dennis C, Elliott MR. A multisite study of health professionals' perceptions and practices of family-centered care. J Fam Nurs. 2002; 8(4): 408–429

[45] Ekberg K, Grenness C, Hickson L. Addressing patients' psychosocial concerns regarding hearing aids within audiology appointments for older adults. Am J Audiol. 2014; 23(3): 337–350

[46] Ekberg K, Meyer C, Scarinci N, Grenness C, Hickson L. Family member involvement in audiology appointments with older people with hearing impairment. Int J Audiol. 2015; 54(2): 70–76

[47] Grenness C, Hickson L, Laplante-Lévesque A, Meyer C, Davidson B. Communication patterns in audiologic rehabilitation history-taking: audiologists, patients, and their companions. Ear Hear. 2015; 36(2):191–204

[48] Meyer C, Barr C, Khan A, Hickson L. Audiologist-patient communication profiles in hearing rehabilitation appointments. Patient Educ Couns. 2017; 100(8):1490–1498

[49] Watts Pappas N, McAllister L, McLeod S. Parental beliefs and experiences regarding involvement in intervention for their child with speech sound disorder. Child Lang Teach Ther. 2016; 32(2):223–239

[50] Damschroder LJ, Aron DC, Keith RE, Kirsh SR, Alexander JA, Lowery JC. Fostering implementation of health services research findings into practice: a consolidated framework for advancing implementation science. Implement Sci. 2009; 4 (1):50

Chapter 4

Planning a Patient- and Family-Centered Approach to Service Delivery

4 Planning a Patient- and Family-Centered Approach to Service Delivery

Carly Meyer, Nerina Scarinci

Abstract

Historically, speech–language pathology and audiology services have been delivered using a traditional mode of service delivery encompassing individual, in-person face-to-face assessment and intervention. Over time, however, the range of service delivery options has expanded exponentially and this chapter will explore each of these service delivery options within a patient- and family-centered framework. Specifically, this chapter will focus on working with other professionals, as well as both in-person and telepractice clinician-delivered services. For each of these models of service delivery, there are a number of different factors that need to be considered when delivering patient- and family-centered care.

Keywords: patient-centered care, family-centered care, service delivery, interprofessional practice, telepractice

Learning Objectives

In this chapter student speech–language pathologists and audiologists will learn the following:
1. The importance of working with other professionals to deliver high-quality patient- and family-centered speech pathology and audiology.
2. How to make clinician-delivered in-person services more patient- and family-centered.
3. How to make clinician-delivered telepractice services more patient- and family-centered.

4.1 Introduction to Planning a Patient- and Family-Centered Approach to Service Delivery

As speech–language pathologists and audiologists, it is common to work within a number of different service delivery models. For each of these models of service delivery, there are a number of different factors that need to be considered when wanting to maintain patient- and family-centered care (PFCC). Most importantly, as a patient- and family-centered clinician it is important to provide your patients and their families with a choice of service delivery, such that the type of service delivery

utilized is driven by patients and their families and incorporates their biopsychosocial needs, preferences, and context. The type of service delivery offered by speech–language pathologists and audiologists should also be flexible over the continuum of care and responsive to families' ever-changing needs.

While historically, speech–language pathology and audiology services have been delivered using a traditional mode of service delivery encompassing individual, in-person face-to-face assessment and intervention, over time, the range of service delivery options has expanded exponentially and in this chapter we will explore each of these service delivery options within a patient- and family-centered framework. In Chapter 6 of this book, we will then describe how speech–language pathologists and audiologists can apply the principles of PFCC to clinical services, across all types of service delivery.

4.2 Working with Other Professionals in Patient- and Family-Centered Care

Before considering the range of service delivery options available for speech–language pathologists and audiologists when planning a patient- and family-centered service, it is important to be mindful that any service provided to patients with communication disability and their families should never be conducted in isolation. It is of utmost importance that we draw on the expertise outside our professional area for the optimal management of the patients and their families. This is where clinicians need to consider working with other professionals as part of a PFCC team, be it a multidisciplinary, interdisciplinary, or transdisciplinary team.

4.2.1 Approaches to Working with Other Professionals

There are a number of subtle differences between multidisciplinary, interdisciplinary, and transdisciplinary practice in health care. In multidisciplinary teams, patients and family members receive care from two or more professional groups independently. Although each professional focuses primarily on his or her area of clinical expertise, he or she does strive for a coordinated approach to care.[1] In interdisciplinary teams, on the other hand, there is greater recognition of the overlap in the expertise and clinical skills between professional groups and thus there is more communication and interaction among team members. Nevertheless, clinical services usually continue to be assigned based on each professional's expertise.[2] Finally, in transdisciplinary teams, clinical services are not divided based on disciplinary expertise, rather, each team member has a responsibility to address the overall functioning of patients. In this way, multiple clinicians of different professional backgrounds come together to provide a joint service, inclusive of assessment, goal setting, and intervention, with the specific role of each team member being dependent on the primary area of concern.[2] This does not necessarily mean that multiple team members are present during each session with patients and their families, rather, one team member is often designated to be the primary provider who is responsible for developing an effective relationship with the patient and his/her family. The primary provider also serves as the key point of contact between the patient and family and other members of the team, and is primarily responsible for maintaining good team communication.[3]

Importantly, depending on the needs, stage of life, and setting, a range of teams involving health professionals can either enhance or negatively impact the patient's and family's experience of care. Jacki Liddle, an occupational therapist in Australia, has provided two case studies for you to work through (see "Student Activity 4.1"). We encourage you to first reflect on the type of team approach that was used with each patient and his or her family, and second, consider how teams can maximize the way they work together to provide PFCC.

4.2.2 Transdisciplinary Teams

Transdisciplinary teams stand out as being the most patient- and family-centered of all approaches and therefore warrant further discussion in this practical guide to PFCC. This is clearly demonstrated in ▶ Fig. 4.1, which has been adapted from Karol[2] who proposed a continuum of team models to illustrate the balance between different levels of professional integration and the extent of patient- and family-centeredness across multi-, inter-, and transdisciplinary approaches.

One of the key reasons why transdisciplinary models of health care are considered to be the most patient- and family-centered is because they allow different health professionals to simultaneously address the patient's biopsychosocial needs by breaking down traditional professional boundaries.[4] The consideration of patients' biopsychosocial needs helps close the gap between health care and daily living,[2] through more holistic goal setting and the promotion of a shared vision among team members.[5] The way in which these boundaries are dissolved in transdisciplinary practice is through role release, which is perhaps one of the most challenging yet important aspects of transdisciplinary team work. In fact, teams only become truly transdisciplinary when team members "let go" or "release" their traditional discipline-specific role. For role release to occur, however, team members must openly share their expertise, and develop trust in the skills, knowledge, and experiences of others in the team.[3] Importantly, within a PFCC model of practice, role release

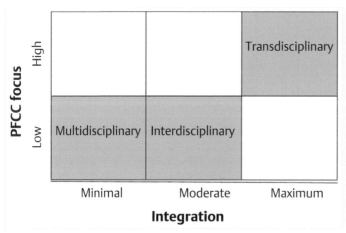

Fig. 4.1 Health care team grid, representing level of integration and extent of person- and family-centered focus. (Adapted from Karol.[2])

Jacki Liddle, Occupational Therapist, Australia

Applying Teamwork to a Rehabilitation Setting

Below is a case study involving Brett, who is about to commence an outpatient rehabilitation program after having a traumatic brain injury. Read the case study and then answer the questions below.

Brett is planning with his team at the hospital how he can return home after a traumatic brain injury. Now that he has left the acute part of the hospital, the team has set up individual appointments for Brett to meet with each of the health professionals who are likely to be involved in his rehabilitation. His family is welcome to attend the appointments, but there are several different appointments, all at different times of the day, and it is proving difficult for Brett's family to get to all of them. Brett is not sure what each of the health professionals do, but is glad to be able to express what his goals are and what he thinks needs to happen in order to return home. After the first of these appointments, Brett wonders if he is doing something wrong. When he mentions the things he wants to achieve, like getting taxi vouchers, and learning how to speak more clearly on the phone so that he can return to work, he is directed by the health professional to speak to the other people in the team about that. He is not sure who in the team does what and is annoyed after the first health professional redirects him into a cooking session in the therapy kitchen.

Questions for Consideration

1. Is Brett receiving a multi-, inter-, or transdisciplinary approach to service delivery?
2. How could the team work differently to provide a more patient- and family-centered service to Brett and his family?

Now that you have had a chance to reflect on Brett's experience working with different health care professionals, the following case presents an alternative approach to team work. Read the case study and then answer the questions that follow.

Malcolm has not driven since he had a stroke and this has placed strain on his household particularly his wife, Sue, who does not drive. Malcolm's primary aim of attending day hospital therapy is to return to driving, so that he can return to work and support his household. If he cannot return to driving, he is concerned that he and Sue may need to move house. He is working with his occupational therapist and physiotherapist on performance components of driving. He is also working with his speech–language pathologist on challenges related to his aphasia. When the team determines together that Malcolm's current performance indicates he is likely to pass a driving assessment, he is referred for an occupational therapy assessment.

Unfortunately, he performs poorly and is not able to complete the full on-road assessment. The team asks to meet with Malcolm, his wife, and the driving assessor to explore the reason for the performance difficulties and reshape therapy goals and approaches. Malcolm and his wife express their distress at the probability that Malcolm may not return to driving and strongly indicate their desire to continue to focus on return to driving as a goal.

During the meeting, it becomes clear that Malcolm found the communication aspect of the assessment particularly challenging and admits that, in addition to the language difficulties he has as a result of aphasia, he is increasingly having difficulty with his hearing. He was unable to attend and follow the verbal instructions given, but was able to control and maneuver the vehicle safely. The driving assessor suggests that lessons may help with confidence and learning to manage the communication aspects of driving. The speech–language pathologist also offers to train the driving instructor and driving assessor and Sue in communicating with Malcolm so that his driving rather than his aphasia can be assessed, and so that communication during driving does not affect his driving safety. After taking the advice of the team, Malcolm also attends an audiology appointment with his wife and as a result is fitted with bilateral hearing aids. Following this process, Malcolm is able to return to driving.

Questions for Consideration

1. Is Malcolm receiving a multi-, inter-, or transdisciplinary approach to service delivery?
2. How is Malcolm's team working differently to Brett's team to provide a more patient- and family-centered service?

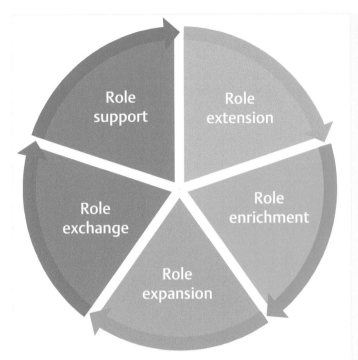

Fig. 4.2 Process of role release. (Adapted from King et al.[3])

also relates to the patient and his or her family, such that the patient and family are fully integrated into the team.[2,3] Karol[2] suggests that transdisciplinary teams are the ones who find it easiest to truly embrace patients and their family members as genuine members of the team.

Role release is a cyclic process (▶ Fig. 4.2) whereby team members participate in several shared learning experiences,[3] as detailed below:

- Role extension: Team members participate in staff development to enhance their theoretical knowledge and clinical skills in discipline-specific areas.
- Role enrichment: A process where information on discipline-specific terminology and evidence-based practice is shared in order to develop a shared awareness and understanding of each other's discipline.
- Role expansion: An exercise where members from each discipline share ideas and information on how they observe and make clinical decisions.
- Role exchange: Team members can formally exchange roles once they have learned the theories, methods, and processes of each others' disciplines.
- Role support: Team members provide ongoing support and advice to one another, particularly when patients and/or interventions are complex and thus require additional skills of the primary provider.

Once the team has successfully progressed through the cycle, it is only then that true role release can occur. Thus, role release should be considered both an action and an outcome. The complexity of role release should not be underestimated as health professionals may need to release their role to others at the same time as taking on other roles.[3] In order to ensure that individual professionals have the skills and expertise to carry out high-quality transdisciplinary practice, professional bodies expect speech–language pathologists and audiologists working in a transdisciplinary team to have undertaken additional training and credentialing in their workplace, which is supported by the phases of role release.[6] As such, student speech–language pathologists and audiologists, as well as recent graduates, are not expected to be able to participate in transdisciplinary practice without mentorship and additional training.

4.3 Clinician-Delivered In-Person Services

Despite there being considerable evidence in support of different models of service delivery, the traditional clinician-delivered in-person model of service delivery continues to be the most common type of service provided by speech–language pathologists and audiologists. These clinician-delivered in-person models of service typically include individual, clinic-based services; individual, mobile services; and group services.

4.3.1 Individual Clinic-Based Services

Individual clinic-based services can take place in a range of settings, including, private clinics, community-based clinics, early-intervention centers, in-patient and out-patient hospital clinics, and rehabilitation centers. Although the extent to which PFCC can be practiced in these settings varies, the provision of individual services has some clear advantages for promoting PFCC, especially for developing an effective therapeutic relationship between the patient, family, and clinician. However, it is important to be mindful that services conducted within a clinical setting inherently create an artificial context that may limit the patient's ability to demonstrate his or her functional capacity and generalize intervention gains into his or her everyday settings. Therefore, when working in a clinic-based service, the onus is on the clinician to ensure that his or her assessment and intervention are tailored to the patient's and family's biopsychosocial needs so they are able to incorporate the strategies learnt from clinic-based services into everyday communication situations.

Student Activity 4.2: Providing PFCC in an In-Patient Hospital Setting

As discussed above, the extent to which you can apply PFCC may vary depending on your particular workplace setting. One environment that clinicians report having more difficulty implementing PFCC is the in-patient hospital setting. Where this setting has traditionally focused on a patient's biomedical needs, an increasing number of hospitals worldwide are adopting more patient- and family-centered practices. You are a speech–language pathologist or audiologist working in an acute hospital setting. As a patient- and family-centered clinician, write down five strategies that you would use with patients and families to promote PFCC.

Within individual clinic-based services, it can also be easy to fall into the trap of presenting yourself as the expert and delivering the intervention to the patient, rather than being a patient- and family-centered clinician who encourages the patient and their family to be the drivers of their own care. Cindy Smith, a speech–language pathologist, who works with young children and their families, discusses how different adult learning styles may impact the way you support and educate family members when using the traditional individual clinic-based model of service delivery (see box on next page "A Word from a Clinical Expert: Addressing Adult Learning Styles in Individual In-Clinic Services").

Although the contribution from Cindy Smith was written in the context of pediatric, clinic-based speech–language pathology services, it is important to acknowledge the role of adult learning styles in empowering patients and families to drive their own care across all clinical contexts and service delivery models, including both adult and pediatric speech–language pathology and audiology services. Below, you will be encouraged to think about how you might ensure your clinic-based speech–langauge pathology or audiology service for Emily and her boyfriend Hugh, who you were introduced to in Chapter 1, is patient- and family-centered.

Student Activity 4.3: Making Clinic-Based Services Count in the Real World

As Emily's speech–language pathologist or audiologist, you regularly see Emily in your clinic to address her voice or hearing difficulties. Although Emily has reported that she is satisfied with these in-clinic services, you can't help but wonder if she is applying the strategies you are discussing in your in-clinic sessions, to her everyday life. In pairs, discuss how you might ensure that your in-clinic service is relevant and is resulting in real-world outcomes for Emily and Hugh.

Overall, individual, clinic-based services have the advantage of allowing you to work one-on-one with the patients and families you care for, and therefore, potentially makes it easier for you to develop an effective patient–family–clinician therapeutic relationship and provide individualized services. However, in order to ensure that your in-clinic services are driven by patients and families and are relevant

Cindy Smith, Speech-Language Pathologist, Australia

With the increasing emphasis in early intervention on empowering the people who are most important in a child's life, speech–language pathologists must focus on helping families become effective facilitators of their child's communication development. This requires a shift away from traditional clinican- and child-centered service delivery to family-centered care. In this model, rather than working directly with the child, the clinician works with the family members to give them the tools they need to help their child.

Working with the child's family involves helping them learn new skills. This requires speech–language pathologists to be cognizant of the principles of adult learning and be aware that different family members will have different learning styles. The types of questions families ask will provide insight into their preferred learning styles. For example, parents commonly ask the following questions:

- **Why** is this information important for me and my child and **why** are we working on these particular strategies?
- **What** is the key information I need to know on this topic?
- **How** do I implement this in real life?
- **What if** this doesn't work with my child?

The adult who asks lots of **why** questions has a learning style that requires a clear rationale for learning, prior to taking on new information. **"What"** questions indicate a learner who needs a lot of information, before being able to implement change. **"How"** questions suggest they learn best by putting the strategy into practice and getting feedback on it, prior to using the strategy independently at home. People who need to work through how the strategy will be used independently of the speech–language pathologist being present may also ask **"what if..."** questions.

If adults' preferred learning styles are addressed effectively in your individual clinic-based services, families are more likely to:

- Be receptive to learning and applying new information.
- Try out what they are learning.
- Enjoy the learning experience—and so, hopefully, come back for more!

When working with families, there are steps to go through to ensure that services match their biopsychosocial needs, preferences, and context. This context includes their learning style. For families who have a **"why"** learning style, the speech–language pathologist needs to encourage them to think about why they are working with the clinician to improve their child's communication. In this step, it is important to first find out what they already know or have already experienced in relation to facilitating their child's communication development. For families who have a **"what"** learning style, speech–langauge pathologists need to provide them with sufficient information, so whatever is being taught is able to be implemented. This contrasts adults who have a different learning style who only require small chunks of information. It can be easy to fall into the trap of lecturing families, but this should be a discussion, finding out what the family feels will be most important, acknowledging their goals, and building from this knowledge. For families who ask lots of **"how"** and **"what if"** questions, it is always useful for the family to try out new strategies with clinician support, before they try it independently at home.

Importantly, when utilizing clinic-based services, it is essential that families continue to work on the strategies they have learnt in clinic at home to help promote carryover into their everyday activities. In order to do this, families always need a clear plan, and writing it down generally helps as a reminder for the family to do something. Before families leave your clinic, you should always make a point of discussing the following:

- What strategies do you feel will be important to focus on at home and how do you think your child will respond if you use these strategies?
- In what situation(s) will you try out these strategies at home?
- How will you remind yourself to use the strategies at home?
- What if the strategies don't go according to the plan?

Finally, what families try out at home will form the basis for the start of the next clinic-based session you have with them, and in fact, will take up a significant portion of the next clinic-based session. Ensure the family knows you will be discussing how the strategies went at the next session.

Gordy Rogers, Speech–Language Pathologist, United States

Pediatric speech–language pathology services can be delivered in a variety of settings, from hospitals and outpatient clinics, to schools and homes. Home-based services boast a number of clear advantages to other settings. They can enable families, the primary stakeholders in the therapy process, to have direct involvement in the day-to-day intervention. Also, in certain client populations, such as those aged birth to 3 years, home-based services are often the preferred setting. And beyond this, home-based services may have advantages in cost-effectiveness for certain clinical service delivery models and in convenience for families. Despite their clear utility, home-based services also come with their own unique set of considerations, and even challenges. In order to maximize the power of this service delivery setting, it's important for all involved to come prepared. The following suggestions, drawn from extensive clinical experience, serve to provide a guide for clinical best practices.

Make a schedule and stick to it. Children are creatures of habit. Routine is one key way that children wrap theirs heads around the world, so to speak. So, as much as possible, it's often best to schedule home-based therapy sessions in a particular time slot (or slots) each week. Your client will come to anticipate the session(s) and be a more receptive participant in therapy. As a practical consideration, clinicians also benefit from committing to a regular home visit schedule rather than providing home services on an ad hoc basis. The same would also apply to follow-up, parent-driven activities outside of direct intervention. Where possible, encourage parents to stick to a schedule. This consistency will foster a stronger commitment from the family and often help yield meaningful clinical results. As long as the clinician provides the example, parents will often follow.

Plant the seed before every session. In the vein of promoting consistency and commitment, encourage parents to inform the child that the clinician will soon be arriving, approximately 10 to 15 minutes before each session. This will pique the child's expectations and simply get him or her better primed for the session. Also, I suggest that parents do their own "warm up" right before the clinician is scheduled to arrive. This can take the form of sitting down with the child, on his or her level, and getting into a play activity with the child. And this play need to take only a few minutes. That is usually all the children would need to get warmed up. Often, when the clinican arrives, the child will naturally bring the clinician into the existing play narrative and the transition to your session then becomes seamless.

Create a play/work space. As any parent can attest, finding a clutter or distraction-free work or play space for your sessions isn't that easy. However, it's a good idea to either prep parents to do so or for the clinician and the family to even spend a few minutes in the first session creating such a space. Pick a place in the home that is not a high-traffic area and is meaningful for that particular family. Make sure it's not too cluttered as it is really important for there to be minimal distractions in the immediate environment.

Parents should actively participate. As tempting as it may be for families to see the time with the clinician as a chance to get the laundry done or to catch up on phone calls or emails, it would be doing the child and the therapy process a disservice to not have parents or caregivers actively involved in sessions in the home. When families play an active role, the clinician is able to impart much more information and strategic suggestions *during* the session. This is lost somewhat if the clinician and family only just chat about it at the end of the session.

Home visits can be wonderfully natural and highly effective means to achieve lasting change in a child's speech and language development. Although they are not without their own inherent challenges, these can be quite easily mitigated by incorporating some of the above strategies. Preparing yourself as the intervening clinician and preparing parents as vital partners in therapy can add real value to the therapy process. The benefits to the child's longer-term life prospects can be immeasurable.

to the patients' and families' biopsychosical context, you might need to be congizant of your own communicative interactions and the environment in which you work (see Chapters 2 and 3).

4.3.2 Individual Mobile Services

In recent years, speech–language pathologists and audiologists have increasingly been providing mobile services to patients' homes, workplaces, and educational settings. This move has been in response to patients' needs and acknowledges the value of providing services in naturalistic settings rather than clinical settings, which are inherently artificial. These ecologically driven mobile services promote learning within meaningful, everyday contexts and enable speech–language pathologists and audiologists to work with others in achieving functional goals.

Mobile services have many obvious advantages to patients and family members and these align with the principles of PFCC. First, by visiting patients in their day-to-day environments, greater access is given to their family members and significant others, including relatives and other important people in their life such as educators, colleagues, and friends. Second, given that patients and family members are often more relaxed in their day-to-day environments, it can be easier to develop effective therapeutic relationships with all those involved, and may result in assessments that are more representative of their true functioning. This is especially true for pediatric patients, who may be more likely to open up and demonstrate their true abilities and, if old enough, share how their communication disability is impacting their everyday life, if they're in a familiar environment (e.g., at home or school). Finally, providing services within the patient's and family's day-to-day life also provides opportunities for discussion around their personal interests and endeavors. In Chapter 3, there was a discussion of the potential benefits of using personal artifacts of the clinician in the clinical setting in order to build effective patient–family–clinician therapeutic relationships. Naturally, within a patient's everyday environment there will be a plethora of artifacts which can be used in rapport building as well as during therapeutic activities.

Given the intimate nature of home visits in particular, there are a number of considerations the clinician must be aware of prior to the first visit, especially if the home visit is your first in-person face-to-face encounter with the patient and their family and you are a relative stranger in their home, workplace, or educational setting. Gordy Rogers, a

speech–langauge pathologist in the United States, shares some key considerations for the delivery of mobile speech–language pathology services (see box on previous page "A Word from a Clinical Expert: Getting Ready for Your Home Visits").

Like there are unique considerations for conducting speech–language pathology and audiology services in the home environment, there are also considerations for conducting these mobile services within the educational system. Speech–language pathologists and audiologists working with school-age children in this setting commonly describe the complexities associated with practicing PFCC. Rebecca Armstrong, a speech–langauge pathologist in Australia who works in an educational setting, shares her thoughts on how PFCC can be facilitated within schools (see box on next page "A Word from a Clinical Expert: Implementing PFCC in an Educational Setting").

> ## Student Activity 4.4: Providing PFCC to Andrew in the School System
>
> You are currently working as a speech–language pathologist or audiologist in an early intervention setting. Your patient, Andrew, will be starting school next year and therefore you have started thinking about transitioning Andrew's care to the educational setting. Given that you are currently practicing in a patient- and family-centered way, and would like Andrew and his family to continue receiving services in this manner, what steps would you take with the school-based team to ensure a successful transition?

4.3.3 Group Services

Another commonly used model of service delivery for patients with communication disability and their family members is group services. Groups can take many forms, including patient groups (e.g., aphasia groups, stuttering groups, hearing impairment groups, school-age language groups, phonological awareness groups), combined patient and family groups (e.g., educational programs, early language play groups, Parkinson's disease groups), education and training groups for parents, spouses, caregivers, and other professionals (e.g., communication partner training, parent education groups), and patient and family run groups. In this latter form, your role as a PFCC clinician might be

A Word from a Clinical Expert: Implementing PFCC in an Educational Setting

Rebecca Armstrong, Speech–Language Pathologist, Australia

We know from this book so far, about the importance of tailoring assessment and intervention to the patient's and family's biopsychosocial needs. For clinicians working with school-age children in educational settings, however, there are a number of additional factors that need to be considered when providing PFCC.

The first factor which should be considered for speech–language pathologists and audiologists working within education is the model of service delivery utilized within this sector. Unlike other models of service delivery where families bring their child to the clinician for scheduled appointments, within the education setting, speech–language pathologists and audiologists see the child while they are attending school. This often means that there is less direct involvement of families in this process. In addition, clinicians working within the educational setting in Australia are often itinerant, meaning they are often spread across a number of schools, and therefore only visit certain schools for set period of time, often without having a strong physical presence at any one school in particular. The nature of this model of service delivery, coupled with the increasingly busy schedules of families, can create challenges for clinicians and families to work closely together. One way to overcome these challenges is for the therapist to be flexible and proactive in modifying the mode of delivery in response to individual family circumstances. This often means advising families when their child will be seen at school, offering additional face-to-face meetings (before or after school, or during school hours), and liaising with families about their communication preferences (e.g., contact via phone, email, or letters sent home to the parent). Another way of involving families in the therapeutic process is to deliver services that aim to reach all those within the school community. This can include utilizing systems already in place within the school, such as building families' knowledge and skills around communication through articles in the school newsletter, or offering parent training sessions outside of school hours.

For clinicians working within the educational setting, there are additional components to consider beyond working with the child's immediate family. While a strong focus on the child's home and working with families remains important, emphasis must also be placed on consideration of the child in the context of his or her educational environment. Indeed the concept of "family" must also extend to include educators and other professionals working within the educational setting. These professionals can range from learning support teachers, to special education teachers, teacher aides, guidance officers, behavioural support staff, occupational therapists, physiotherapists, and even speech–language pathologists from other agencies (and the list could go on!). This increased emphasis on the child in the context of his or her classroom and the broader definition of "family" means school-based speech–language pathologists and audiologists must instil as part of their everyday practice, shared decision making not only with parents, but also with the entire school team. In this way, in addition to building strong relationships with the students and their families, it is paramount for school-based speech–language pathologists and audiologists to build effective and therapeutic relationships with the entire school team. Working alongside educators also allows clinicians to understand the demands placed on teachers and other professionals in the classroom setting, and allows for the sharing of knowledge and skills to help optimize the child's capacity for learning and success at school. Therefore, despite there being challenges in the implementation of PFCC within educational settings, the rewards and benefits reaped by employing a PFCC approach are far-reaching.

to initially facilitate the establishment of a group based on the psychosocial needs, preferences, and contexts of your patients and their family members, but then not attend in person leaving the running of the group to the patients and their family members.

The benefits of group therapy in a PFCC context are numerous. For example, both patients and family members can receive emotional and practical support from others going through similar experiences, and can share important insights and learnings from the perspective of patient and family members. These two mechanisms of patient and family support are key components of PFCC. Similarly, by learning from one another, there is a greater focus on active problem solving rather than clinician-directed care, which in turn promotes the patient and family as experts in their own care and

Linda Worrall, Speech–Language Pathologist, Australia

Aphasia is a family problem. The sudden impact of a stroke sends shockwaves through the family. When someone has aphasia, it is very difficult for him or her to comprehend what has happened through a haze of impaired language. Family members often have many questions as it is unlikely that they have heard of aphasia before. The Aphasia Language Impairment and Functioning Therapy (LIFT) program at The University of Queensland, Australia, creates a therapeutic environment that allows the person and his or her family to comprehend the effects of aphasia, adjust psychologically and emotionally, as well as improve their communication for everyday life.

The key ingredients of LIFT are the inclusion of family in the program, the emphasis on achieving relevant communication goals for the person with aphasia, as well as the strong and relatively intensive dose of evidence-based one-to-one therapy (48 hours over 8 weeks), group therapy, and computer sessions. A major strength of the program is that LIFT is for a cohort of people with aphasia and their families. One cohort starts and finishes the program together, creating group cohesion. The reported outcomes of the program as a whole include a sense of achievement, confidence, and greater self-esteem. These are achieved through more rapid language gains, more communicative opportunities, and more social connectedness for both the patients and their families during and after the LIFT program.

For some people with aphasia and their family members participating in the LIFT program, this may be the first time they have met other people with aphasia and their families. The LIFT schedule not only enables clinician-directed conversations about life with aphasia in group therapy, but also creates multiple opportunities for people with aphasia and their families to rediscover social connectedness in the waiting area as well as over coffee or lunch. By including families starting their journey with aphasia as well as families who have lived with aphasia for many years, there is a wealth of family experiences the group can share that ultimately provides hope and an overall sense that family life with aphasia can be good.

An illustration of how LIFT puts the patient in the driving seat of therapy is the "*the final celebratory challenge day*" on the last day of the program. On the challenge day, people with aphasia have the opportunity to show their extended family members how far they have progressed with a "challenge task" they have worked on during the program. The challenge task aims to not only stretch and extend the person's communication skills, but also aims to give them the excitement of achieving something that they didn't think they could do. On the final day, all participants with aphasia present their challenge task with family and friends. Friends and family are frequently amazed and very proud that their family member with aphasia could achieve the task and are often emotional if the task is a rediscovered skill. Challenge tasks have included showing and instructing the audience on how to bake a lemon slice, composing and performing a song with a guitar, and recreating an occupational role by training the audience to tie knots.

Patient-centeredness and family-centeredness does not just mean that families are included or that relevant goals are set. The therapeutic relationships must also be enacted in a respectful but authentic way. LIFT aims to develop strong relationships among all therapists, participants with aphasia, and their family members. Therapists model supported communication strategies, and conversation partner training is a group therapy session. LIFT seeks feedback from all participants (including family) from each cohort, so that the program uses a continuous quality improvement cycle. Consistent use of active listening, small talk, nonverbal connections (e.g., eye contact, reassuring pats on the arm), and humor plays a role in ensuring that all families with aphasia feel included and valued in the group.

Quality of health care can be viewed in terms of structures, processes, and outcomes. LIFT aims to provide a quality patient- and family-centered aphasia program. The structures that enable this include a language assessment and goal setting session before LIFT begins, an invitation to family to attend the program, a schedule that allows for clinician-directed and nondirected interactions, and therapists who can model supported communication strategies. The processes that enable this are the waiting room chats, the structured group sessions that discuss matters such as social connectedness, and embedding the challenge day task throughout the program as a motivating tool. Outcomes include measured and self-reported communication gains across the ICF, high satisfaction ratings, and greater social connectedness.[7]

The challenge for families with aphasia is to find a way to maintain and sustain the gains made through LIFT without the ongoing need for clinician input. A greater network of community aphasia groups would help as would a greater proliferation of self-management tools via telerehabilitation. In the meantime, and until we can improve in this area we know that participants with aphasia and their families are getting a "lift" through the LIFT package of evidence-based practices.

subsequently facilitates self-management. Kylie Webb, a speech–language pathologist in Australia, has directly observed the benefits of parent groups in intervention for young children with language delay and she shares these experiences in **Video 4.1**. In particular, she notes how parents can help one another in their awareness of the positive role they can play in their child's communication development. One particular strategy you can use to empower the groups to solve their own problems is to turn any patient and family member questions back to the group for others' perspectives, rather than answering these questions yourself.

Working with patients and their families as a group also facilitates more holistic intervention through providing opportunities to apply therapeutic strategies to functional situations (i.e., the participation domain of the International Classification of Functioning, Disability, and Health [ICF]). Providing group services has the additional advantage of possibly being a more cost-effective option for patients, families, and clinicians, which may make them a more viable option for some patients and families, and potentially, more appealing to health system managers or business operators. Perhaps one of the best ways to highlight the benefits of providing in-person groups in speech–language pathology and audiology is to hear from experts in the field who share their experiences about the benefits of group services, not only for patients with a communication disability but also for their family members. The first contribution from Linda Worrall, a speech–language pathologist in Australia, discusses the benefits of group intervention for patients with aphasia and their family members (see box on previous page "A Word from a Research Expert: Patient- and Family-Centered Care in the Aphasia LIFT Program"). The second contribution, from Jill Preminger, an audiologist in the United States, contains a reflection on how group services can be used within an adult audiology rehabilitation service (see box on next page "A Word from a Research Expert: Reflections on Providing Aural Rehabilitation Groups for People with Hearing Loss and Their Family"). For audiologists, many useful resources for running groups for adult patients with hearing impairment and their families are available from the Ida Institute (www.idainstitute.com).

In-person group services clearly have a number of advantages for providing PFCC; however, as both Linda and Jill aluded to, this type of approach comes with some inherent challenges. Other challenges might be that clinicians find it more difficult to cater for the individual needs of each patient and family member. This is particularly relevant for speech–language and audiology services where you need to consider the impact of the communication disability itself on the capacity of patients to participate fully in this more complex communication scenario.

> **Student Activity 4.5: Facilitating Patient and Family Involvement in Group Sessions**
>
> Imagine for a moment that you are a clinician who is running a group for people with Parkinson's disease. Shane and Lorna are in your group. Given that Shane has a soft, breathy voice and Lorna has a hearing loss, how will you facilitate their active participation in the group?

Clinician skills for running group services: It is clear that, in order to provide effective group services, clinicians need to draw on a different skill set to what they would normally during individual clinic-based services. Ultimately, a good group facilitator needs to be skilled in helping the groups meet their goals. These skills might come easier to some than others, depending on your own experiences; however, these skills are essential if you are to deliver patient- and family-centered education and training. The qualities that adult learners have indicated they value in a group facilitator include warmth, indirectness, good content knowledge, honesty, good communication skills, flexibility, and enthusiasm.[9,10] We have provided a checklist in ▶ Fig. 4.3 that you can use to ensure you are doing all you can, as the facilitator, to help engage patients and families in groups.[11]

Another important consideration when facilitating group education and training sessions is how diversity among members of the group manifests in group dynamics. A well-known model of group interaction, developed by Lacoursiere,[12] summarizes the phases a group can go through in developing and establishing an effective and productive group. The phases of this group life cycle are summarized in ▶ Fig. 4.4. In the "forming" stage, a group comes together with diverse needs, expectations, and backgrounds and thus is initially dependent on the facilitator to clarify the objectives and ground rules for the group. In this first phase, it is important that group members get to know one another such that they can recognize the shared knowledge and expertise each member brings to the table.

A Word from a Research Expert: Reflections on Providing Aural Rehabilitation Groups for People with Hearing Loss and Their Family

Jill Preminger, Audiologist, United States

Several years ago, I was doing research measuring the efficacy of group aural rehabilitation (AR). I was interested in learning what content was the most valuable. To accomplish this, I ran some groups in which participants practiced communication strategies, other groups in which participants performed auditory/visual speech perception exercises, and other groups in which participants worked on training tasks as well as psychosocial exercises (as a way to promote support from peers). In the midst of running these AR groups, I gave a presentation about the project at our local hearing loss support group, Hearing Loss Association of America, in order to recruit research participants for the AR groups. During the question and answer session one of the people in the audience asked me "What about the spouses?" I asked her to explain what she meant and she said "Spouses are affected by hearing loss, we need to participate in groups too." I was momentarily dumbstruck, as I had never read any literature about including spouses in the AR process—after the fact, I learned that there were a few articles on this topic, but I had never seen it or read it! Her statement amazed me because it made so much sense. Of course, spouses are impacted by hearing loss! Of course, spouses should be included in the AR process! The next week I started to design a new project in which we ran AR groups for patients with hearing loss on their own and other groups in which patients attended with a family member (mostly spouses). Several years later when I analyzed the data across all of these studies, I found that varying the content in AR group made little impact on outcomes. However, the presence of a family member makes a very significant impact on outcomes. Patients who attended AR groups with their family had much larger improvements in self-reported hearing disability as compared to patients who attended AR groups on their own.[8]

I learned three important lessons while running AR groups that I want to share. First, scheduling the groups can be very difficult. Getting five couples into a meeting room, at the same time, for four separate sessions used to take days of phone calls—perhaps today it would be easier with online scheduling systems like Doodle Poll? Second, facilitating AR groups is very easy. Once, we had everyone in the room, all the facilitator had to do was bring up a topic (e.g., what's the most difficult thing about living with hearing loss?) and participants immediately began to share their experiences. One person would tell a story and another would share a similar story. A spouse would share an awkward experience and other spouses nodded their heads and laughed. The group members reveled in their commonalities, and the mutual support was evident to all. The third lesson is one that I am currently exploring. I have been running focus group interviews in which we have been discussing what to include in online AR groups. Because scheduling the groups is so difficult, I would like to see if we could move them to the internet. In these focus groups, we have been discussing content to be included. After sitting around the conference table and discussing the experience of living with hearing loss, many have voiced concerns about achieving the same experience online as in person. At the end of the group, a few have asked, "Can we come back and meet again?" or, "Can you invite me to your next group?"

Future research will have to determine if the same benefits exist when participating in internet-based AR groups as compared to in-person AR groups. However, what we know now is that patients and their families benefit from, and enjoy, participating in AR groups. I have also learned that leading AR groups is an ideal way to provide family-centered care. When participants find commonalities in their lived experiences, they feel understood and validated, by both the other group participants and the facilitator. These findings suggest that holding AR groups in a clinical setting can be difficult to schedule but extremely worthwhile. Facilitating AR groups for patients and families is an easy and enjoyable way to promote trust, provide empathy, and improve outcomes.

	You have used the three basic principles of group facilitation:
	You have brought out the perspectives of all group members
	You have focused on how people participate in the process, not just on what gets achieved
	You don't take sides
	You encouraged participation:
	You made sure that everyone feels comfortable participating
	You have developed a structure that allows all contributions to be heard
	Members feel good about their contributions
	The contributions and direction of the group discussion is driven by the group, not the facilitator
	No one is criticised for their contributions
	You consider the communication needs of all group members and make the necessary adaptations to the environment
	As a facilitator, you:
	Understand the objectives of the group
	Introduce an ice-breaker activity, including group introductions
	Develop and maintain ground rules with all members of the group
	Keep the group and the discussion moving forward, while at the same time, being adaptive and flexible
	Involve everyone in the discussion
	Sensitively manage conflict
	Present information clearly and logically
	Demonstrate good active listening by reinforcing what group members have said

Fig. 4.3 Group facilitation checklist (Adapted from Community Tool Box.[11]).

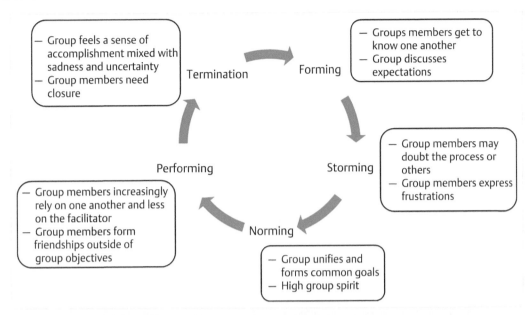

Fig. 4.4 The life cyle of groups.[12]

The Parkinson's disease group you are running with Shane and Lorna is a new group involving four couples who have not previously met. Brainstorm ideas for how you could foster the development of the group in the "forming" stage, such that the group members can understand each other's biopsychosocial needs, preferences, and context.

After the group has formed together, "storming" among group members will inevitably occur as differences emerge in expectations and reasons for being there. Group members may also question the objectives of the group and potentially even you as the group facilitator. It may be confronting for you as the group facilitator if a group member appears defensive or angry, but it is important to remember not to take this personally and realize that this is a normal process that occurs when groups come together. This tension in group dynamics sometimes needs to be addressed on an individual basis, but nonetheless, may still result in a group member leaving.

Consider how you might manage the storming phase of the Parkinson's disease group with Shane and Lorna. There is one member in particular, whom you have not met before, who is being very defensive, and at times, displays his frustration at why he is there when he doesn't believe he is benefiting from the group.

Approximately halfway through the group program, "norming" will occur. In the norming phase, you will sense the group coming together and working cooperatively toward common goals. After coming through the storming phase, you will finally see an improvement in the spirit and collegiality of the group. Now knowing the group better, some planned activities may need to be tailored to the individual dynamics of this group. At this stage, it is important to keep in mind that no two groups will ever be the same!

The forth phase of a group life cycle is "performing." At this time, you, as a group facilitator, play less of a role as the individual group members have more confidence and trust in one another.

You are still needed, however, and play a key role in encouraging autonomy, providing feedback, and continuing to encourage group members to share what they have learned.

The final phase of group dynamics is aptly called "termination." At the end of any group program, where friendships may have formed and a codependence on peers for support and growth has developed, it is essential that you, as the group facilitator, provide an opportunity for the group to experience closure.

Student Activity 4.8: Promoting Closure in Groups

What group activity might you plan to promote closure at the termination phase of your Parkinson's disease group?

It is clear that in-person speech–language pathology and audiology services offer many advantages to providing a patient- and family-centered approach to service delivery. At times, however, you may be working with patients and/or families who do not live within reach of an in-person service. Therefore, as a patient- and family-centered clinician, you may need to consider offering your service via telepractice.

4.4 Clinician-Delivered Telepractice Services

Telepractice is a growing model of service delivery in speech–language pathology and audiology. Internationally, telepractice is defined as the use of telecommunication technology to provide assessment, intervention, consultation, and/or supervision in speech–language pathology and audiology by linking clinicians to patients, families, and other professionals who are at a distance.[13,14]

Telepractice has long been promoted as a way of increasing access to speech–language pathology and audiology services to patients and families across their life span. Traditionally, telepractice was seen as an option only for those people who were living remotely and unable to access services in their local area. More recently however, speech–language pathologists and audiologists have started to recognize the benefits of using telepractice for all patients and families, including those who live in large metropolitan cities. In fact, some research suggests that telepractice may even lead to more patient- and

family-centered interactions. First, as telepractice takes place in the patient's own home, workplace, or educational setting, it inherently allows for consideration of the patients' and families' biopsychosocial context. In this way, telepractice facilitates the provision of patient- and family-driven care. Second, because the interaction occurs in each person's own space, the power balance between the patient and the clinician is equalized, and the patient has more control over the interaction.[15] This results in patients accepting more responsibility for their role in the interaction, and hence requires more effortful communication, greater patient participation, and more patient- and family-driven care.[16] Third, telepractice can promote the development of a more effective patient–family–clinician therapeutic relationship, as distance and the use of technology necessitates the slowing down of communication interactions. This is accomplished through more overt turn-taking processes and both parties paying closer attention to social cues.[17] For these reasons, telepractice has been observed to result in patients, families, and clinicians becoming more invested in the therapeutic relationship.[18] Monique Waite, a speech–language pathologist in Australia, describes the ways in which telepractice can promote PFCC (see box on next page "A Word from a Research Expert: Benefits of Telepractice for Promoting Patient and Family-Centered Care").

4.4.1 Types of Telepractice

Telepractice can take one of three forms: (1) synchronous; (2) asynchronous; or (3) a hybrid approach. Synchronous telepractice is the most commonly used form of telepractice and refers to the real-time interaction between a clinician and a patient and his or her family. Synchronous telepractice most typically occurs through the use of videoconferencing software, including the use of specialized equipment, licensed programs, and/or freely available software such as Skype and FaceTime. Of all the forms, synchronous telepractice is the one that most closely resembles traditional in-person services, in that the patient, family, and clinician are interacting in real time, albeit at a distance. On the other hand, asynchronous telepractice refers to a delayed clinical interaction, whereby clinical information is shared via the internet, most commonly by email and through internet clouds and portals, but there is no real-time contact between the patient, family, and clinician. The types of clinical information exchanged can include images, videos, test results, written information,

Monique Waite, Speech–Language Pathologist, Australia

Families and clinicians working with young children with hearing and communication disorders have reported many positive ways that telepractice has been used to promote a patient- and family-centred approach to care.

Telepractice offers the perfect opportunity to provide intervention within the child and family's natural communication and social environment. Activities can be built around communication with who and what is in the child's natural environment, including extended family members and friends, toys, pets, and hobbies. Practicing in the home environment facilitates carryover of skills. There is also the opportunity to assess the child's communication within the natural environment and make observations to identify family needs such as support with behavior management. The family can feel more comfortable by being in the home and not having to travel long distances to a clinic: *"After a while you actually become almost like a fly on the wall since the parents get so used to it. You almost see a side of them and behaviors from them that you wouldn't see if they were in a center."* (speech–language pathologist)

Telepractice can be used to support the whole family. Through technology, other family members can also attend the session from any location. Similarly, other professionals and services can be brought in to support the family's needs. Videoconferencing, online groups, and e-learning can provide family education and connect families for peer support: *"I know as a parent I was really lost when [child] was first diagnosed. This is something I was really craving because I felt I didn't have anyone else to chat to about it. Now it's great because there's a whole heap of like-minded parents in the same [online] group."* (Parent)

Telepractice can be used to develop the family's strengths. With young children, families need to take on more responsibility in a telepractice session as the clinician is not physically in the room. However, this presents the perfect opportunity for the clinician to coach the families to support their child's communication developent. This empowers families, building their confidence and skills: *"I really love when I see parents just take it on. And they are absolutely the expert in what their child should be doing. And that's exactly how it should be."* (Teacher of the deaf)

Telepractice can provide access to services in a way that is responsive to the family's needs. It allows access to more frequent and specialized services than may be available in the family's local area, enabling families to choose a service that best meets their biopsychosocial needs and preferences. Telepractice is not just for rural families; it can also meet the needs of urban families that might have difficulty getting into the clinic. A flexible approach may involve providing a hybrid service of both in-person and telepractice sessions, with telepractice being used on the occasion of bad weather or illness. Finally, scheduling of telepractice sessions can be more responsive to the family's needs, for example, it may be easier to schedule sessions early in the morning, as there is no need to travel: *"Overall for me it fills a gap that we couldn't have filled locally and I'm glad that we've been able to access it despite the fact that on paper I thought we looked like we had access to a lot of things, but they weren't relevant."* (Parent)

In telepractice, the patient–family–clinician relationship is critical. Clinicians and families who use telepractice highlight the importance of preparing the family's expectations for how the telepractice service and sessions will run and of taking the time to identify the family's needs, build rapport, confidence, and trust. As the family may play a greater role in the session than in traditional intervention, it is essential that the family members are adequately prepared and supported to do this, for example, through providing them with resources and technical support: *"I've found the first few sessions are really important to build up the relationship and rapport and build up the trust. I just listen to their needs, see what they want, and then quite often, what I want to give is not what they want."* (Teacher of the deaf)

A Word from a Research Expert: The Clinical Application of Hybrid Telepractice

Annie J. Hill, Speech–Language Pathologist, Australia

Meet Ben and Julia, a couple aged in their mid-seventies. Ben had a stroke 10 years ago which resulted in moderate physical difficulties and moderate language difficulties (aphasia). Ben had aphasia rehabilitation soon after his stroke but hasn't engaged in any therapy for about 7 years. While Ben and Julia live in the city, Ben's mobility difficulties mean that he can only get to a speech–language pathology clinic if Julia drives him. Ben is keen to engage in more aphasia therapy. Ben, Julia, and the speech–language pathologist discussed a variety of service delivery options and agreed a hybrid model of telepractice would best enable PFCC for them. Using synchronous telepractice, Ben and Julia videoconference with a speech–language pathologist from their home once a week, and between these sessions Ben engages in personalized therapy tasks on an iPad. His progress through these tasks is monitored and updated remotely by the speech–language pathologist (asynchronous telepractice). Using the synchronous telepractice model, Ben and Julia can both attend the session with the speech–language pathologist, thus including Julia in Ben's sessions and enabling the clinician to observe their communication patterns in their home context. By remotely monitoring Ben's progress through the therapy tasks delivered on the iPad, the speech–language pathologist is able to observe which tasks Ben is finding more challenging or those that are too easy. The asynchronous telepractice connection enables the speech–language pathologist to change the tasks in a timely manner, that is, there is no need to wait for the next videoconferencing session to update the tasks.

To trial the hybrid telepractice service delivery approach, Ben's language skills and his quality of life were formally assessed both before and after the period of therapy. Ben and Julia also reflected upon their perceptions of telepractice in an interview at the end of the trial. The therapy was delivered over two, 4-week blocks, with an interval of about 3 months in between. The synchronous telepractice sessions were done using a software-based videoconferencing system on an iPad. The asynchronous telepractice therapy was accessed by Ben using an iPad, while the clinician accessed the system on his or her desktop computer. Based on the initial assessment results, the speech–language pathologist fully customized therapy tasks for Ben across the areas of naming, comprehension of sentences and paragraphs, repetition of complex words, reading functional words, and spelling. Full customization included choosing target words that were meaningful to Ben and Julia, such as family members' names, foods regularly prepared, and places visited. The synchronous telepractice sessions were designed around communication partner training and addressing any other communicative goals that arose for Ben and Julia.

Ben engaged in intensive therapy practice using the iPad across both blocks of therapy. He averaged a total of 76 min/d of therapy in Block A and 97 min/d in Block B using asynchronous telepractice. The eight synchronous telepractice sessions lasted 50 minutes each and Julia attended each of these. Overall, Ben made improvements across all areas of communication, with his greatest improvement in reading comprehension, naming, and picture description. With regard to quality of life measures, Ben showed improved quality of life after therapy Block A, with further improvements in the area of participation after therapy Block B. Satisfaction with the hybrid telepractice service delivery model was measured using a five-point (5 = yes, definitely so; 1 = no, definitely not) aphasia-friendly survey. Ben was highly satisfied across all items and reported that he especially valued being able to do the therapy at times and places that suited him, usually in the comfort of his own home and that he could take a break when he needed to. Ben also reported that it was easy to find the time to do the therapy because of the flexibility that asynchronous telepractice enabled. He valued the in-built feedback so that he knew instantly how he was progressing. Ben and Julia both said that they enjoyed the synchronous telepractice sessions with the speech–language pathologist. Julia learnt a few new communication strategies and revised some strategies she had been using to enhance the communication between her and Ben. Ben reported that he enjoyed seeing the speech–language pathologist who was designing tasks for him and that he had the opportunity to give her feedback on the tasks in terms what he felt was working best for him and others that were too easy or too difficult. Both Ben and Julia said that they would like to use telepractice again and would recommend using it to others with aphasia as a way of facilitating PFCC.

A Word from a Research Expert: Increasing Talk Time for People with Aphasia using Asynchronous Telepractice

Caitlin Brandenburg, Speech–Language Pathologist, Australia

The Communicative Fitness program is a behavioral intervention which aims to increase the amount of language practice by people with aphasia in their everyday lives. Increased speech output aims to improve verbal language impairment by capitalizing on principles of neuroplasticity, as well as stimulate social participation.[19] The program uses CommFit, a smart phone app paired with a wearable monitoring device (i.e., accelerometer), used to measure how much a person is talking.[20] Much like wearable devices that measure the number of steps you take in a day, the CommFit technology works as a "pedometer for language"—a simple measurement device that gives the user constant, easily interpretable feedback on the amount of language practice. Incorporated in the app are goal setting and feedback elements. The program can be used as a form of asynchronous telepractice alongside traditional language therapy (hybrid telepractice), or as a self-management tool, although it is recommended that there is some oversight by a speech–language pathologist or other trained health professional. This oversight ensures that the program is appropriate for the individual (e.g., not appropriate for Wernicke's aphasia, where the person with aphasia already speaks in long sentences that are jargonistic, and thus the production of words is not the concern) and that the goal talk times are set at a level that is therapeutically appropriate, and does not cause harm due to vocal overuse. Early results have indicated that users with aphasia are able to increase their talk time, improvements were shown on language and psychosocial measures, and the program was rated highly.[20]

As communication by its very nature includes another person, the success of the Communicative Fitness program relies on meaningful involvement of both the patient with aphasia and his or her family to motivate behavior change. Some patients in pilot studies increased their talk time by humming, talking to themselves, or doing individual therapy tasks. Although these behaviors should not be discouraged, the practice task should be as close as possible to the behavior to be improved to best stimulate neuroplastic change. Thus, practice of real-world conversations, with all their intricacies, should make up the bulk of the talk time measured by the app. When beginning the program, a person with aphasia may attend sessions with his or her family member, who is educated about the program alongside the patient. With support from the speech–language pathologist, the family member may take this information and set up regular calls or visits with each of their adult children for speaking practice, possibly setting topics to guide these interactions (e.g., talk about the news, talk about a TV show after each week's episode). Ideally, the conversation would be meaningful to motivate a lengthier one and thus maximize language improvement through the principle of salience.[19] Depending on individual patient and family needs, preferences, and contexts, some individuals will be highly motivated by the feedback elements of the app, while others may prefer in-person guided therapy. Prescription of the program in a PFCC rehabilitation model should take this into account.

Development and evaluation of the Communicative Fitness program and technology for people with aphasia present an interesting case study on the nexus between application of neuroplasticity principles, mobile technology, self-management, and PFCC.

and resources. Finally, hybrid services involve a combination of synchronous, asynchronous, and/or in-person services. Importantly, hybrid approaches may involve any combination of the above services, but not necessarily all three.

In many clinical situations, hybrid telepractice is the preferred solution, and is the form of telepractice, which is increasingly being adopted by speech–language pathologists and audiologists. In this chapter we share two contributions from research experts who have experience in using sychonous and asynchronous telepractice in a patient- and family-centered context. First, we hear from Annie J. Hill, a speech–langauge pathol-

ogist in Australia, who describes the clinical application of hybrid telepractice and how it promotes patient self-management and PFCC (see box on previous page "A Word from a Research Expert: The Clinical Application of Hybrid Telepractice"), and then we will hear from Caitlin Brandenburg, another speech–language pathologist in Australia, who developed an asynchronous application of telepractice for people with aphasia, and who describes how it can be used in conjunction with in-person speech–language pathology services in order to promote PFCC (see above).

Where the above methods of telepractice described by Annie and Caitlin involved the provision of individual telepractice services to patients and their families, there is emerging evidence that group services can also be delivered via telepractice. Below, Rachelle Pitt and Annie J. Hill, both speech–language pathologists in Australia, share their experiences from running PFCC groups for people with aphasia via telepractice.

Rachelle Pitt and Annie J. Hill, Speech–Language Pathologists, Australia

Did you know there is emerging evidence that patients with aphasia and their family members benefit from group services delivered via telepractice? Usually, group telepractice would involve using multipoint videoconferencing software with screen sharing functionality so that all participants can connect into the group, see each other, and interact with therapy resources. In a recent study, 19 patients with aphasia accessed 12 weeks of group therapy via telepractice from their home. Three to four patients with aphasia accessed each 1.5-hour session via their own internet connection or mobile internet hotspot. Following treatment, these participants and seven family members participated in semistructured in-depth interviews and completed a satisfaction survey. Findings confirmed that delivery of aphasia group therapy via telepractice is feasible and results in improvements in communication-related quality of life. For example, one person with aphasia said *"it's amazing the difference it makes over only a couple of weeks."* Both the patients with aphasia and their family members appreciated being able to meet others *"in the same boat"* and helped them to feel like they weren't alone in their journey of recovery. Some patients with aphasia felt like they had a *"new family"* in the group. Despite connectivity issues, participants were satisfied with telepractice technology and felt that telepractice saved time and money, and was easier to access from home. Family members felt that telepractice was convenient for them and helped the patient with aphasia to be more independent. All participants would recommend the telepractice group to others.

The above contributions provide only three examples of how telepractice has been successfully used with patients and families in order to promote PFCC. In order to ensure the successful implementation of telepractice, however, you need to consider a number of additional factors at play, relating to the patient, their family, and you as the clinician.

4.4.2 Patient and Family-Related Factors Impacting Telepractice Services

Patient- and family-related factors impacting telepractice services include their communication, physical, and sensory abilities; cognitive and behavioural functioning; attitude toward telepractice; and, their access to resources.[14] Clearly, there are certain communicative, physical, and sensory abilities that may impact the success of a telepractice mode of service delivery. These include receptive and expressive language skills, literacy skills, speech intelligibility, hearing impairment, visual impairment, manual dexterity (e.g., the impact of arthritis on the patient's ability to use a mouse and keyboard), and the patient's and family member's ability to stay seated from a long period of time. Cognitive and behavioral skills such as attention and concentration, as well as the presence of any cognitive impairment, may also influence a patient's or family member's ability to actively engage over telepractice. A person's attitude toward telepractice should also be considered as you should not assume that all patients and family members will perceive telepractice positively. Lastly, the patient's access to the resources required to conduct telepractice must be considered, including the availability of necessary technology and devices, internet connection, and a quiet working space, as well as access to appropriate training and support in how to use telepractice.[13,14]

In order to practice as a patient- and family-centered clinician, you will need to not only identify the factors that may influence the success of a telepractice model of service delivery, but also work with the patient and their family to overcome any possible barriers. Importantly, in collaboration with the patient and the family, you may find that certain forms of telepractice are more suitable for one patient over another, and it might be that you need to reflect and modify the service as you progress through intervention.

4.4.3 Clinician-Related Factors Impacting Telepractice Services

Just as there are patient- and family-related factors to consider in telepractice, there are also factors relating to you, the clinician, which must be considered. In fact, the clinician's attitude toward telepractice is a key factor influencing the adoption and success of telepractice. It has long been assumed that in-person speech–language pathology and audiology services are the gold standard, with telepractice being considered by some as inferior and only something you would consider if in-person services are not possible. This attitude largely stems from fear that it is not be possible to develop an effective therapeutic relationship between the patient, family, and clinician using telepractice.[21] However, research has found that the majority of clinicians who hold this view have not had direct experience in the delivery of teleservices and therefore this attitude is largely unfounded.[22] As described earlier, telepractice is associated with a number of benefits for patients and families, one being the promotion of even greater levels of PFCC, relative to in-person services.

Another key consideration when delivering speech–language pathology and audiology services via telepractice is your role as a clinician in developing an effective patient–family–clinician relationship. This relationship is initially developed through the clincian's ability to promote a friendly and warm interaction, which in telepractice literature, is commonly referred to as "bond." Bond is frequently linked with "presence," which is often assumed to mean a physical presence, however, this is not necessarily the case. Essentially, if the clinician, patient, and family are able to embrace telepractice and immerse themselves in this virtual space, then this sense of presence can still be strongly felt. However, to be able to engage in a virtual space in this way, factors such as sound and picture quality, synchronization, and distractions need to be addressed. In effective telepractice, patients, families, and clinicians report forgetting that they are not physically present in the same location.[23]

In the same way that "presence" can be maintained in telepractice, so can the portrayal of empathy. However, it must be acknowledged that when delivering a session via telepractice, speech–language pathologists and audiologists need to rely more on verbal communication and less on nonverbal gestures in order to demonstrate empathy. For example, in situations where you as the clinician might normally express empathy through touch, eye contact, and passing a box of tissues, in telepractice, clinicians may need to overcompensate for the lack of physical presence by honing their verbal interaction skills such that they learn to rely more heavily on their verbal emphathetic responses.[24]

Finally, it would not be fair to discuss the application of telepractice in speech–language pathology and audiology without recognizing that clinicians

---

Student Activity 4.9: How Do You Feel about the Use of Telepractice in Speech–Language Pathology and Audiology?

Given that your own attitude toward telepractice might influence your own decision to use telepractice with patients and their families, we encourage you to spend some time now reflecting on your attitude toward telepractice by considering the survey questions below and circling the answer that best represents your attitude[22]:

1. Assessments can be completed as accurately via speech–language pathology and audiology telepractice as compared to in-person assessments.

   strongly agree   agree   neutral   disagree   strongly disagree

2. Rapport between clinicians, patients, and families can be established during speech–language pathology and audiology telepractice as strongly as during in-person services.

   strongly agree   agree   neutral   disagree   strongly disagree

3. Speech–language pathology and audiology telepractice services can be as effective, in terms of patient and family progress toward goals, as in-person services.

   strongly agree   agree   neutral   disagree   strongly disagree

4. I would be interested in providing speech–language pathology and audiology services via telepractice.

   strongly agree   agree   neutral   disagree   strongly disagree

need appropriate training, support, and preparation before considering telepractice as an option for service delivery.[13] Although some clinical services provide specialist training and guidelines for the implementation of telepractice, most commonly, it is individual clinicians who initiate the introduction of telepractice, and therefore are responsible themselves for adequately preparing for telepractice and for troubleshooting on the job. Monique Waite, a speech–language pathologist in Australia, has provided five top tips to help clinicians prepare for telepractice (▶ Fig. 4.5).

Choose equipment to meet your needs	• Invest in equipment with quality and functionality to make the most of your sessions. • Videoconference systems that can be used on multiple platforms, such as the PC, tablet and smartphone offer flexibility for access and enable sessions to be conducted anywhere. • A web camera with zoom functionality and a visualiser or document camera may be helpful to you.
Prepare the clinic and home environment	• Work with the family to set up the most appropriate space. • A defined space will enhance child engagement and ensure privacy. • Good acoustics, lighting, and the elimination of visual distractions are essential.
Address expectations and etiquette	• Discussing telepractice practicalities and expectations for family involvement ahead of time will help the family feel prepared. • There is certain telepractice etiquette that needs to be considered and discussed with the family, including explicitly asking if your communication partner can see and hear you, announcing who is in room but not in shot, announcing if you are going to mute yourself, and asking permission to record the session. • Also, given that a patient- and family-centered telepractice session is going to involve more than two people, and nonverbal communication, particularly eye contact, can be difficult to read, it is really important to address people by name so that it is clear who the message is being directed too.
Be prepared	• Sessions need to be planned ahead of time so the family can prepare resources. • Consider using duplicate or complementary resources to facilitate interaction. • Ensure access to appropriate support personnel and have a back-up plan in case of technology failure.
Make the most of your sessions	• Facilitate the interaction between the patient and family member through modelling and coaching. • Be creative and make the most of the family's environment, for example by taking the session outside with the use of a smartphone or tablet. • Make the most of the technology, including the use of multimedia resources and apps.

Fig. 4.5 Top tips for telepractice by Monique Waite, speech–language pathologist, Australia.

4.5 Summary

In this chapter, we have described different models of service delivery in speech–language pathology and audiology and how these can be patient- and family-centered. In whatever clinical practice setting you find yourself, you should consider the information and clinical examples in this chapter and apply the tips and suggestions provided to optimize PFCC. It is most likely you will work at least initially in a traditional clinician-delivered in-person service; however, it is also highly likely that your practice will expand to include mobile services, group services, and telepractice over time. Such services are rapidly growing in popularity and acceptance with patients and their families and it is important that speech–language pathologists and audiologists are responsive to this and that they apply PFCC principles in these new models of service. Finally, in this chapter, we describe multidisciplinary, interdisciplinary, and transdisciplinary practice, the latter being not only the most challenging model for health professionals, but also the one that has the potential to be the most patient- and family-centered.

4.6 Reflections

Please respond to the following reflection questions in your PFCC journal:

1. What are the differences between multidisciplinary, interdisciplinary, and transdisciplinary health care practice?
2. What are the phases of group dynamics you should be aware of when running speech–language pathology or audiology groups for patients and families?
3. Consider a recent clinical encounter in speech–language pathology or audiology. How could telepractice have been applied in that encounter for the patient and/or his or her family? Were there elements of the traditional appointment (or before or after it) that could have been provided via telepractice?

References

[1] Turnerstokes L, Nair A, Sedki I, Disler PB, Wade DT. Multidisciplinary rehabilitation for acquired brain injury in adults of working age. Cochrane Database Syst Rev. 2005(3):CD004170

[2] Karol RL. Team models in neurorehabilitation: structure, function, and culture change. NeuroRehabilitation. 2014; 34(4):655–669

[3] King G, Strachan D, Tucker M, Duwyn B, Desserud S, Shillington M. The Application of a transdisciplinary model for early intervention services. Infants Young Child. 2009; 22(3):211–223

[4] Smits SJ, Falconer JA, Herrin J, Bowen SE, Strasser DC. Patient-focused rehabilitation team cohesiveness in veterans administration hospitals. Arch Phys Med Rehabil. 2003; 84(9):1332–1338

[5] Davies S. Team around the child: working together in early childhood intervention. Australia: Kurrajong early intervention service; 2007

[6] Speech Pathology Australia. Transdisciplinary Practice: Postition Statement. 2014. https://www.speechpathologyaustr alia.org.au/SPAweb/Members/Position_Statements/spaweb/Members/Position_Statements/Position_Statements.aspx?hkey=dedc1a49-75de-474a-8bcb-bfbd2ac078b7. Accessed March 15, 2019

[7] Rodriguez AD, Worrall L, Brown K, et al. Aphasia LIFT: exploratory investigation of an intensive comprehensive aphasia programme. Aphasiology. 2013; 27(11):1339–1361

[8] Preminger JE, Meeks S. Evaluation of an audiological rehabilitation program for spouses of people with hearing loss. J Am Acad Audiol. 2010; 21(5):315–328

[9] Clark JI. Who, Me Lead a Group? Seattle, WA: Parenting Press Inc.; 1984

[10] Brundage DH, Mackeracher D. Adult Learning Principles and Their Application to Program Planning. Toronto, Ontario: Minister of Education; 1980

[11] Community Tool Box. Chapter 16. Group facilitation and problem-solving. http://ctb.ku.edu/en/table-of-contents/leadership/group-facilitation/facilitation-skills/checklist. Accessed July 12, 2017

[12] Lacoursiere RB. The Life Cycle of Groups: Group Development Stage Theory. New York, NY: Human Science Press; 1980

[13] Speech Pathology Australia. Telepractice in Speech Pathology: Postition Statement. 2014. https://www.speechpathologyaustralia.org.au/SPAweb/Members/Position_Statements/spaweb/Members/Position_Statements/Position_Statements.aspx?hkey=dedc1a49-75de-474a-8bcb-bfbd2ac078b7. Accessed March 15, 2019

[14] American Speech-Language-Hearing Association. Telepractice: overview. http://www.asha.org/Practice-Portal/Professional-Issues/Telepractice/. Accessed June 20, 2017

[15] Simpson S, Bell L, Knox J, Mitchell D. Therapy via videoconferencing: a route to client empowerment? Clin Psychol Psychother. 2005; 12(2):156–165

[16] Day SX, Schneider PL. Psychotherapy using distance technology: a comparison of face-to-face, video, and audio treatment. J Couns Psychol. 2002; 49(4):499–503

[17] Jerome LW, Zaylor C. Cyberspace: creating a therapeutic environment for telehealth applications. Prof Psychol Res Pr. 2000; 31(5):478–483

[18] Bischoff R, Hollist C, Smith C, Flack P. Addressing the mental health needs of the rural underserved: findings from a multiple case study of a behavioral telehealth project. Contemp Fam Ther. 2004; 26(2):179–198

[19] Raymer AM, Beeson P, Holland A, et al. Translational research in aphasia: from neuroscience to neurorehabilitation. J Speech Lang Hear Res. 2008; 51(1):S259–S275

[20] Brandenburg C, Worrall L, Copland D, Rodriguez A. An exploratory investigation of the daily talk time of people with non-fluent aphasia and non-aphasic peers. Int J Speech-Language Pathol. 2017; 19(4):418–429

[21] May J, Erickson S. Telehealth: why not? Perspectives of speech–language pathologists not engaging in telehealth. JCPSLP. 2014; 16:147–151

[22] Tucker JK. Perspectives of speech–language pathologists on the use of telepractice in schools: quantitative survey results. Int J Telerehabil. 2012; 4(2):61–72

[23] Simpson SG, Reid CL. Therapeutic alliance in videoconferencing psychotherapy: a review. Aust J Rural Health. 2014; 22 (6):280–299

[24] Porcari CE, Amdur RL, Koch EI, et al. Assessment of post-traumatic stress disorder in veterans by videoconferencing and by face-to-face methods. J Telemed Telecare. 2009; 15(2):89–94

Chapter 5

**Identifying Patient and Family
Member Needs through
Assessment**

5 Identifying Patient and Family Member Needs through Assessment

Louise Hickson, Tanya Rose, Nerina Scarinci, and Carly Meyer

Abstract

When practicing as a patient- and family-centered clinician, core to the entire assessment process is the importance of asking patients and families about what they hope to achieve from your speech–language pathology or audiology service, and ensuring that you identify both patient and family strengths as well as challenges. This chapter will discuss how patients and families can be involved as partners in the entire assessment process, including preassessment planning, case history taking, observation, self-report, formal assessment, and interprofessional assessment. This chapter will also focus on how speech–language pathologists and audiologists can share assessment results in a patient- and family-centered way. A key skill underpinning all assessment processes is the use of effective patient- and family-centered communication, and as such this chapter will focus on applying some of the knowledge discussed in Chapter 2. A range of patient- and family-centered resources are presented.

Keywords: patient-centered care, family-centered care, assessment, diagnosis, patient- and family-centered communication

Learning Objectives

In this chapter, student speech–language pathologists and audiologists will learn the following:

1. How to involve families in the assessment of adults and children with communication disability?
2. Strategies for effective patient–family–clinician communication during assessments.
3. The importance of preassessment planning and the interactions you might have with patients and families prior to an assessment appointment.
4. The value of observations of patient and family as part of the assessment process.
5. How to use patient and family self-report measures to gain insight into the everyday impacts of communication disability?
6. Effective ways to discuss assessment findings with patients and their families.

5.1 Introduction to Identifying Patient and Family Member Needs through Assessment

"One of the most sincere forms of respect is actually listening to what another has to say."

(Bryant H. McGill)

In Chapter 1, you were introduced to the World Health Organization's International Classification of Functioning, Disability, and Health (ICF) framework[1] (see ▸ Fig. 1.2) that encourages speech–language pathologists and audiologists to consider all aspects of a person's life that will impact on their functioning and disability. Core to the entire assessment process is the importance of asking patients and/or family members about what they want from the assessment and your service and to keep in the forefront of your mind that the assessment should be as much about identifying patient and family strengths as it is about identifying patient and family communication challenges. According to Hebbeler and Rooney,[2] assessment should include the following:

- Involve patients and families as full partners in the assessment process.
- Provide you, the clinician, with information about the patient's and family's biopsychosocial functioning based on multiple sources.
- Provide information to guide intervention.

In this chapter, we will discuss how to involve patients and families as partners in the assessment process, and how you can use multiple sources to obtain information about the patient's and family's biopsychosocial functioning. In Chapter 6, we will discuss how you can use the information obtained from a patient- and family-centered assessment to guide intervention. Before we get started, we would like you to reflect upon your own experience as a patient or family member in a health care setting. It's always good to put yourself in the patient's shoes so as a future speech–language pathologist or audiologist you can "*do to others as you would have them done to you.*"

Think about a health care assessment that you have experienced as either a patient or family member where you were happy with the outcome. It is possible to be happy with the appointment even when the news from the clinician is not good? For example, you received an unexpected diagnosis. What made this experience feel right?

Now, think about a health care assessment that you have experienced either as a patient or family member where you were not completely happy. What was it about that experience that bothered you?

5.2 Involving Patients and Families as Full Partners in the Assessment Process

Effective patient- and family-centered care (PFCC) means that patients and family members need to drive the assessment. Involving families in the assessment process can take many different forms, and the ways in which families are involved are likely to differ according to the setting in which you are working. It is also relevant to recognize that involving families may be more challenging in certain environments. For example, an audiologist who is working in an aged care setting may see a patient for a hearing screening assessment at an aged care facility when their family is not present. Likewise, a speech–language pathologist working in a hospital setting may assess a patient on the ward when family members are not visiting. It is relevant to consider that family involvement extends beyond "face-to-face" contact during a single assessment appointment. Speech–language pathologists and audiologists who are truly endeavoring to identify the needs of the patients and their families should consider how they involve family members who may not be able to attend the face-to-face assessment session(s). Perhaps this interaction could be through a telephone call, Skype call, telepractice platform, or via email, having obtained consent from the patient to do so.

When trying to involve families, speech–language pathologists and audiologists need to state, both verbally and in their written communication, that family members should attend the assessment session, whenever possible. Importantly, you, as the clinician, need to be cognizant of the definition of "family" discussed in Chapter 1 as being "two or more individuals who depend on one another for emotional, physical, or economic support"[3] and be open to involving a broad range of family members in the assessment process. Front of house staff who are responsible for booking patient appointments should invite families to attend appointments. Singh et al.[4] recommend, for example, that front of house staff making appointments could say: "*Our experience is that it is very helpful if you can bring a friend or a loved one along to the appointment. Who would that be?*" If the patient is uncertain and asks why, then the response could be "*There is a lot to discuss and it helps to include family and friends in the process.*" Crais[5] also provides examples of words that can be used to indicate a desire for collaboration right from the first phone call or initial communication with the family. For example: "*We value what you know about your [x]*," "*We want to gather information from you and others important to [x]*," "*We know that you know [x] best so we need your help.*" or "*We will try to figure out together what's best for [x].*"[5]

If working in a setting where you do not always have an opportunity to work directly with family members, ensure that you still explicitly state that involvement from family members is crucial and ensure you obtain information about family members' preferred method of communication. You may need to be flexible in the options you provide and consider that for busy family members, email, for example, may be the preferred mode of communication. Be intentional about asking for patient and family member preferences for information sharing. It may be best to do this when obtaining consent for assessment and consent for you to discuss patient information with persons other than the patient.

Both patients and family members may need to be convinced as to why it is important that family members attend the initial assessment session. This may not be what the patient and family members are used to in their interactions with other health professionals. In addition, it may also mean that family members need to take time off from work and/or reschedule other commitments so that they can attend the assessment appointment. Brainstorm in a small group, possible reasons why it is important that family members attend the assessment session.

When you are face-to-face with patients and families, the most efficient way to ensure that families drive the assessment is to engage in triadic conversation and this is only possible if family members are involved and engaged. Even when family do attend an assessment session, they may remain reluctant to come into the appointment and indicate they will stay in the waiting room. One way to address this situation is to use both the patient's and the family member's names when you call them from the waiting room, for example, *"Shane and Lorna, it is nice to see you both, please come this way."* Another option, if family members continue to indicate they will wait outside, is to take the patient (Shane) into the clinic room first, explain why it would be helpful to include Lorna and seek his permission to invite her into the room. Some younger and older adults, may see the inclusion of family as challenging their autonomy and it is important to make it clear that this is not your intention.

5.2.1 Starting a Patient- and Family-Centered Assessment

Once you have the patient and his or her family in the clinical room, remember to outline what will happen in the appointment and restate how long has been scheduled for the session. It might help some patients to use a visual schedule when communicating this information. It is also important to consider that the order in which you conduct the assessment may differ for different patients and families. For example, when working with adults, the assessment session may start by completing a case history interview with the patient and his or her family; however, for pediatric patients, the assessment may start with an observation of the patient interacting with his or her family member/s. Speech–language pathologists and audiologists need to be flexible in their approach and endeavor to start the assessment in the way that will most assist to put the patient and the family at ease and help to build rapport and engagement.

5.2.2 Optimizing Patient–Family–Clinician Communication

Just as it is important for speech–language pathologists and audiologists to be flexible in their assessment approach, there are some essential communication skills described in Chapter 2 that are also important for developing an effective patient–family–clinician relationship. *"Begin as you mean to go on"* is a famous catch-cry relevant here and is considered a key to success in relationships, business, and in life more generally. Effective relationship building is acknowledged to be crucial for patient and family satisfaction, compliance, and positive outcomes (see evidence for PFCC in Chapter 1). As such, it is vital that you are cognizant of nonverbal, verbal, and written communication strategies that enhance the patient–family–clinician relationship.

While there are numerous ways you can go about establishing effective patient–family–clinician relationships, never underestimate the importance of nonverbal communication strategies (see Chapter 2). For example, maintaining eye contact with patients and families goes a long way to show that you are present. This may mean physically repositioning yourself by "squatting down," or sitting on a chair so that you are at the patient's and family member's eye level.

The quote at the start of this chapter reminds us that, as a clinician, the most important thing you can do in the assessment phase is to listen carefully to what your patients and their families are saying. Chapter 2 details the key elements of effective communication with patients and their families that demonstrate you are listening. Effective listening skills are essential in order for us to appreciate the patient's and family's situation, understand their desires, reach common ground about areas for priority, and facilitate shared decision making.[6]

> ### Helpful Tip: The 7-Second Rule
>
> Remember to wait as long as possible (at least 3 seconds with some experts recommending up to 7 seconds) after you have asked a question for the patient and family to reply.[7] It might help to count 1-and-2-and-3-and etc. in your head. Try not to jump in too soon with more questions.

There are resources available such as the Effective Listening and Interactive Communication Scale (ELICS)[6] to assist you to assess and reflect on your own listening skills. King and colleagues[6] encourage clinicians to consider different types of listening skills in the context of an ongoing and evolving patient–family–clinician relationship. For example, when first meeting a patient and his or her family, you typically need to engage in *receptive listening*, which involves giving mindful attention to acknowledging that patient and family concerns are legitimate, being present in the moment, and listening to what is not said.

In addition to being mindful of your verbal communication during assessments, it is also important to consider the appropriateness of your written communication with patients and families. For example, ensure that all written information, including appointment letters and consent forms, are written at an appropriate readability level (see Chapter 3). Also ensure that there are multiple ways for your patient, who may have a communication difficulty, to contact you, keeping in mind that your patient may not be able to use the telephone to cancel or reschedule an appointment. You may also like to consider including a "photo signature" at the end of any written communication, whereby you include a "headshot" photograph of yourself, along with your name and profession. Many of your patients and their family members may be working with numerous health professionals and a "photo signature" may help the patient and his or her family to get to know you and orient the written information you provide with your service.

Finally, clinicians conduct assessment appointments on a daily basis, but this is very often a novel experience for patients and their families who may not know what to expect and may be feeling a gamut of emotions relating to the assessment session. It is important that you take a moment to put yourself in others' shoes and consider how patients and families may be feeling as the assessment process begins. Also remember that assessment is often an ongoing process and relationships established initially may be fleeting. An effective therapeutic relationship between patient, family, and clinician, one of the key elements of PFCC, is something that needs continuous attention.

Student Activity 5.3: Patient and Family Emotional Responses to Assessment

Brainstorm and then discuss different emotions that patients and family members might be feeling as they commence the assessment process. Refer to the case studies in Chapter 1 and imagine you are:
- Miranda and Flynn attending an initial speech–language pathology assessment for their son Andrew.
- Emily attending an initial speech–language pathology assessment with her boyfriend Hugh.
- Lorna attending an initial audiology appointment with her husband Shane.

Putting yourself in your patient and family member's shoes, how are you feeling about the assessment process?

5.3 Obtaining Information about the Patient's and Family's Biopsychosocial Functioning

It is important to keep the ICF in mind when planning how you will gather information about the patient's and family's biopsychosocial functioning. In speech–language pathology and audiology assessment, it is all too easy to focus on gathering information about the patient's body structure and function; however, you also need to consider how you will gather information about their activity, participation, and other contextual factors that are likely to influence their care. Rebecca Nund, a speech–language pathologist in Australia, explains in **Video 5.1** how you can use the ICF to frame your patient- and family-centered assessments taking into consideration each domain of the ICF. Although this video focuses on a pediatric speech–language pathology example, it has application to all patients and families.

Assessment in speech–language pathology and audiology typically involves gathering information from a range of sources, including preassessment planning, case history, patient and family observation, patient and family self-report, and formal assessment. It is essential that patient- and family-centered clinicians triangulate the information gathered from multiple sources to obtain a complete picture of the patient and his or her family. Triangulation in this context means answering this question: Does the clinical assessment match the self and family reports of real-world performance and match the reports of others, such as teachers, caregivers, and other health professionals?

5.3.1 Preassessment Planning

It is common for patients to attend speech–language pathology and audiology assessment appointments with little preparation. Patients, and families if they attend, also typically do not know what to expect. Crais et al[8] describe 41 family-centered practices in pediatrics, and 17 of these relate to preparing for the assessment which can also apply to adult patients and their families. Some examples are as below:
- Making contact with the patient and family before the assessment.
- Asking the patient and family to identify areas for assessment and what they want to get out of the assessment.

- Asking the patient and family if the patient has been previously assessed, and if yes, how did they feel about the previous assessment.
- What activities or techniques used in the previous assessment(s) were most and least successful and how did they feel about previous assessment results.
- Asking the patient and family to identify strategies that can be used in the assessment.

Before contacting the patient and family about their upcoming assessment appointment, we recommend you consider what helpful information the patient and family can gather prior to their first assessment appointment. This may involve prompting patients and family members to gather information from other key communication partners such as childcare workers, teachers, employers, friends, peers, other family members, and other health professionals. It may also involve sending the patient and/or his or her family a self-report measure to complete. Family members may also be asked to record specific observations related to the patient's hearing and/or communication with familiar and unfamiliar communication partners.

Depending on the specific work setting, speech–language pathologists and audiologists should also consider if it is possible for themselves and/or another team member to meet with the patient and his or her family before the actual assessment session. This pre-assessment planning meeting can be used to gather important background information; explore current communication skills, including communication strengths; talk through different assessment options tailored to patient and family concerns and priorities; and to offer choice for determining the best place and time to gather information about the patient and family. As Crais so aptly asserts, *"It is important to remember that families can only be informed decision makers and actively help plan their [family member's] assessment when they know all options available to them."*[5]

Helpful Tips for Preassessment Planning

Crais[5] lists several example questions which are relevant for both speech–language pathologists and audiologists to consider when conducting a preassessment interview with patients and families:

"What are your concerns and what do you want to get out of the assessment?"

"Do you prefer a more formal (e.g., describing properties of typical standardized tests) or informal (e.g., describing more informal measures) assessment approach?"

Prelock and colleagues[9] suggest other preassessment questions for family members including the following:

"What about [your family member] brings you joy?"

"What are you most worried about?"

"What have you been told about [your family member]?"

"How would others describe [the patient's] strengths and challenges?"

"What is your expectation for this assessment?"

After asking patients and families to complete any pre-assessment tasks, it is important that once you meet with them, you remember to follow-up on any information you have asked patients and families to gather. For example, if you have asked patients and/or family members to complete a self-report questionnaire, it is vital that at some stage during the assessment session you ask for this information and pay due attention to the information provided. It can be extremely frustrating for patients and families, and also damaging to the patient–family–clinician relationship, if they have spent time compiling this information and the speech–language pathologist or audiologist does not ask for this information; or if they do ask, they do not give appropriate attention to the information by commenting or asking further questions, and/or do not explain how the information will be used.

Take a moment to look back at the cases introduced in Chapter 1—Emily, Shane, and Andrew.

Emily is due to come and see you for an audiologic review after having been diagnosed with a hearing loss 6 months ago. Emily is finding it increasingly difficult to cope in her university studies and has started to withdraw from social situations with her friends because she finds it difficult to communicate in noisy places. Work in small groups to discuss how you would help Emily and her boyfriend Hugh prepare for the appointment.

Think back to when Shane and Lorna came for their initial speech–language pathology assessment appointment. When Lorna made the appointment, she mentioned that they were having a lot of difficulty at home because Shane's speech was rapidly deteriorating. Work in small groups to discuss how you would help Shane and Lorna prepare for the appointment.

Miranda and Flynn are coming along to see you as part of their regular intervention; however today's focus is a formal assessment of Andrew's school readiness. Andrew is starting school in 6 months, and they are struggling to get him ready for the change in environment and are worried that he won't cope with the demands of school. Work in small groups to discuss how you would help Miranda and Flynn prepare for the appointment.

Speech–language pathologists and audiologists should be aware that there are a number of international institutes and centers, for example, the Ida Institute (www.idainstitute.com) and CanChild (www.canchild.ca) who have developed many useful resources to assist clinicians to deliver PFCC. All materials have been developed by bringing together international experts in the field to collaborate on how to make PFCC a reality and many resources are freely available on their websites for speech–language pathologists, audiologists, patients, and their families to access. For example, the Telecare section of the Ida Institute website (http://idainstitute.com/toolbox/telecare/) has a range of tools designed for pre-assessment planning. Using telepractice in this context is particularly appealing as patients and their families can complete the tools online and email a copy to the clinician prior to attending the assessment appointment. Alternatively, patients and/or families can print out completed tools and bring them to discuss at the appointment.

5.3.2 Taking a Patient- and Family-Centered Case History

After completing any preassessment planning with the patient and family, it will be timely to ensure that you obtain information from a case history interview. Your clinical setting is likely to have a plethora of standard case history forms for you to use with patients and families. However, these standard case history forms traditionally focus on the body structure and function levels of the ICF. In order for your case history interview to be truly patient- and family-centered, you will need to take a broader perspective of the patient's functioning, and obtain information not only about the patients with the communication disability, but also their families. In your case history, consider obtaining perspectives from both the patient and family member regarding their participation in a variety of communication activities which are meaningful for the family. For example, are there particular contexts, be they everyday routines (e.g., family mealtimes), activities (e.g., traveling in the family car), events (e.g., family gatherings), locations (e.g., a favorite family restaurant), or family communication partners (e.g., siblings, adult children) where communication is particularly challenging or particularly successful? If you have the resources available to do so, the case history interview may also provide an opportunity to ask patients and families if they would like to connect with another family in a similar situation.

Patients and family members can find it frustrating and tiring to continually repeat "their story" and provide detailed demographic information time and time again with each and every encounter with a health professional. You may like to consider resources such as CanChild's "The Kit: Keeping it Together" (www.canchild.ca/en/research-in-practice/the-kit-keeping-it-together), which is a tool to assist parents to organize information when they are interacting with numerous different service providers and systems. The Kit, for example, contains forms to assist parents to document personal information about their child and also their child's likes and dislikes, which can then be provided to various health professionals.

When asking questions in your case history, you must pay particular attention to the types of questions you ask. The types of questions should vary according to the communication skills of your patients and their families, keeping in mind that some family members may also have a hearing loss and/or other types of communication disability. Typically, case history–taking questions should be open-ended in nature in order to encourage patients and their families to speak freely. As a patient- and family-centered clinician, it is important to elicit the patient's story (see Chapter 2). There may be instances, however, where using closed-ended questions, as a supported communication technique best supports patients and family members to participate in the case history process. You may also need to explicitly state why you are asking some questions.

Some example first questions for the patient may be:

Why have you come here today?
Tell me about your ... hearing/communication with others?
How does this affect you?

Some example first questions for family may be:

Tell me how you see things from your perspective.

What do you think about (patient's name) hearing/communication with others?
How does this affect (patient's name)?
How does this affect you?

In a moment, we are going to ask you to brainstorm some additional questions you might incorporate into your case history in order to capture a broad view of the patient's and family's biopsychosocial functioning. First, however, take a moment to view **Video 5.2** where patients and families have shared how their communication disability impacts them in the community, as this is the type of information that will be important for you to elicit in a patient- and family-centered case history.

Consider again the cases of Emily, Shane, and Andrew. Work in pairs and develop five open-ended questions you would ask the patient and/or his or her family at the start of their assessment appointment. These questions should extend beyond the "standard" case history questions, which typically relate to only basic demographic information, developmental/medical history, etc.

Once you have the list of biopsychosocial case history questions, take turns in role playing the clinician and the patient and/or family member. When acting as the clinician, challenge yourself to do more listening than talking!

Reflect on how you felt as both clinician and patient/family member. Were you comfortable? What was hard and what was easy?

Now that you have had a chance to generate your own biopsychosocial case history questions, read how Lesley Jones, an educator in the United Kingdom, approaches a patient- and family-centered case history interview (see box on next page "A Word from a Clinical Expert: Making a Connection and Completing a Task: Patient- and Family-Centered Consultations in Speech–Language Pathology and Audiology").

A Word from a Clinical Expert: Making a Connection and Completing a Task: Patient- and Family-Centered Consultations in Speech–Language Pathology and Audiology

Lesley Jones, Educator, United Kingdom

At the same time as making a connection with their patient and family members, the health professional has to provide a structure and complete certain tasks. Keeping the flow and the empathy going at the same time as gathering information, processing it, and coming to an agreement with the persons on the receiving end about how to deal with their communication problems requires certain skills. Keeping several things going at once can be learnt and is helped by recognizing what those skills are and being aware of when you are not using them. We do them without thinking a lot of the time, but I've found it helpful to acknowledge them and try them out in teaching and practice. Here's a few ideas from medical education and counseling.

Introductions and preparation

- Introduce yourself, for example, *my name is Mary. I'm a speech–language pathologist/audiologist.* I know it sounds like a support group, but it's necessary, especially accompanied by a friendly professional approach. Finding out what your patient prefers to be called is also useful.
- Establish why they are there and what can be expected, for example, *I'll be mostly talking with Emily (the patient) at first, but I am pleased you are here too, Hugh, and there will be time for both of you to describe your point of view.*

Ways of finding out what is going on

- Start with an open question beginning with how, when, where, why, or what, for example, *what made you come today?*
- Let the patient tell his or her story in his or her own way, for example, *could you tell me a bit about what is happening with your hearing/communication at the moment?*
- Respond to their comments appropriately only after leaving plenty of pauses at the end of their first opening response.
- Give them time to think about their replies and process your comments.
- Note the effect on them of telling their story and acknowledge any distress or anger, for example, *I can see that its upsetting for you to talk about it, but it might help us to try to find a way through it together.*
- Ask similar open-ended questions of family members to understand their story, for example, *why do you think you are both here? What did Emily (patient) tell you about the appointment last time she came?*

What to do with what you've heard

- Internally process the information and sort it in your mind by using some of the following methods.
- If taking notes, explain what you are doing and why, and try not to interrupt the flow.
- Pick up on cues, for example, *so you mentioned a friend who didn't get on with hearing aids—why was that do you think?*
- You may need to follow an open-ended question with a closed one, for example, *how important is the look of the hearing aid to you when you said it was unflattering?*
- If the story has gone off on a tangent, try to pick up a relevant point, for example, *can I take you back to when you said that when you're out with your friends, sometimes they talk to Hugh as though you're not there?*
- Pick up on any nonverbal cues from family and patient, for example, *I notice you raised your eyebrows when Emily said she always looks at you when she's speaking.*
- Clarify what you think you heard, for example, *so it's worse when there's a lot of people around? Have I got this right ...?*
- Summarize major points, for example, *so you feel that with your University commitments ramping up, it's time to do something about your hearing?*

Set the agenda

- Let the patient and family know what will happen after the case history, for example, *is it ok to do some tests and see where we are at the moment and then talk about some options?*
- Include a time frame if you can, for example, *are you happy if we look at A and B now and leave C until another time?*
- End an appointment with a summary of the current situation and the forward plans for patient and family, for example, *so today we have found that you have a mild–moderate hearing loss, and when we meet next time, we will discuss options to help you with that.*

Importantly, once you have elicited the patient's and family's own story, you may then need to ask some closed-ended questions to obtain factual information and fill in gaps in the history. You could do this by summarizing what you know from what you have heard and then asking some clarifying questions. For example, you may say to Andrew's parents: *"I understand that Andrew has been having some difficulty interacting with his peers at kindergarten. How many close friends would you say that Andrew has now?"* or to Emily *"You said how hard it is for you to cope with your studies when you can't always hear the group discussions in the classroom. Do you have any ringing in your ears that also makes this difficult?"* Another way to obtain this factual information and to potentially save time in the appointment may be to use a case history intake form that the patient and/or family could be asked to complete prior to the appointment as part of your preassessment planning. As a patient- and family-centered clinician, it will be important to include on any case history form a space for patients to record the names and ages (where appropriate) of their important family members and the nature of their relationship (e.g., grandparents, siblings, aunts, uncles, adult children, spouse, partner).

It is also important to consider how you end the case history interview. Invite both the patient and his or her family to ask you questions and to share any additional information that they may want you to know. Also consider that some family members may be looking for strategies and/or things they can do to assist their family member, so be prepared with any practical and helpful information you can provide or things that family members might be able to do in between the end of the session and when you will see them next, for example, recording a communication sample. Also consider if it would help the patient and family to share the information you have obtained with other health professionals involved in their care and gain consent and the necessary details to do so.

5.3.3 Patient and Family Observation

Observations of the patient interacting with family may serve as a cornerstone assessment method in PFCC. Speech–language pathologists and audiologists can not only observe numerous aspects of the patients' communication simultaneously (i.e., hearing, speech, language, voice, fluency, and multimodal communication skills), which can be subsequently analyzed in a variety of formal and informal ways, but importantly, clinicians can also observe the communication interaction between the patient and his or her family, and also the family member's communication skills. Furthermore, you should seek to obtain the most accurate and best sample of the patient's communication skills and it is likely that is going to be better facilitated by observing the patient communicate with his or her family members, compared to a less familiar clinician. The importance of naturalistic speech–language pathology and audiology services was discussed in Chapter 4. Information about both the patient's and family members' communication strengths and difficulties can be obtained from observations captured spontaneously in locations such as the hospital bedside and in the waiting room, or more intentionally, in the clinic room. For those clinicians who work in the acute setting, the Inpatient Functional Communication Interview (IFCI)[10] has been developed to evaluate how patients with communication disorders function in the hospital environment. In Chapter 3, we discussed the importance of setting up the physical environment to promote PFCC. Next are some helpful tips on how you might set up a clinic room to optimize the observational assessment of the interaction between a young child and his or her parent. First, however, hear from Kylie Webb, a speech–language pathologist in Australia, about how she sets up her clinic for a patient- and family-centered assessment (**Video 5.3**).

It is very important to give thought to the room setup. For example:

- Select age-appropriate toys that are likely to stimulate interest from the child; however, avoid making the room "too busy" by, for example, offering too much choice for the child and parent as this may be overstimulating.
- Include some toys/materials that are likely to be familiar for the family (e.g., books, bubbles, blocks, etc.). Entering a clinic room with only "flashy" and expensive toys may make the room less familiar for both the child and parent, particularly if the parent does not know how to use the objects.
- Consider conducting the observation in the child's home environment with toys/materials, which are familiar to all involved, or if unable to do so, suggest that the parent bring a favorite toy/book to the clinic.
- Set the room up in a way that will encourage the child to communicate. Put some objects of interest in the child's level of sight, but out of reach to see if the child asks for the objects. Include objects that the child requires help from the caregiver to operate (e.g., clear containers with tight lids so that the child can see what is inside, but cannot open without assistance; or bubbles with a tight lid that cannot be undone without assistance; or a wind-up toy that needs a parent to operate). Perhaps include some duplicated toy objects (e.g., two toy cars or two small balls), to see if the parent plays alongside his or her child. Consider situating an adult size chair near the toys, to see if the parent sits down on the floor with his or her child (if he or she is able to do so) or observes from the chair. Also consider how you could select objects that might stimulate the child to comment (e.g., having a puzzle with a piece missing or an object that doesn't belong with others such as a sock in the box containing blocks).

Before starting any sort of observational assessment, however, it is important to consider what you will say to the patient and his or her family.

This is a good opportunity to clearly convey (1) that you are taking a strength-based perspective by wanting to observe what the patient and his or her family can do, not only what they cannot do; (2) that you recognize the important role that family members play in communication interactions; (3) that by setting the room up in a family friendly way, the patient and family may feel more at ease and facilitate a more naturalistic assessment.

Importantly, observational assessment is not only restricted to speech–language pathology. Consider how an audiologist could observe a patient with a hearing loss. For example, the audiologist could observe the following:

- Does the patient turn in responses to sound in the clinic environment?
- Does the patient "hear" better when he or she looks at the speaker's face?
- Does the patient misunderstand any questions asked?
- Does the patient let the family member answer all the questions?
- Does the patient move closer to the speaker to hear?

At the end of the observational assessment, consider what you will say to the patient and family. First, you should explicitly ask the patient and family about how they think the interaction went and whether they think it was typical of how they would interact and communicate at home. There can be a variety of reasons as to why the interaction may not be typical, for example, the patient and/or family member may be feeling unwell, tired, and/or anxious. If the patient or family comments that the interaction was not typical, ask them to describe how they consider the interaction to be different.

Finally, although you may still be formulating your professional opinion regarding the observational assessment, in our experience it can be very beneficial to ensure that the clinician makes some positive comments about the interaction and communication observed. This comment should be genuine and honest. It can help to make a positive comment about the interaction (e.g., I noticed that there was a lot of smiling during that play); the child's communication (e.g., I noticed that [child's name] was clearly showing you things that he wanted to play with) and the parent's communication (e.g., I noticed that you used lots of different facial expressions when you were playing with [child's name]).

In this section, we have described how you can perform observational assessment within the clinical environment; however as a patient- and family-centered clinician, it is important to step outside the clinical environment to see how the client functions in other contexts, such as during other health care appointments, in other educational contexts, and during patient and family recreational activities. View another video from Kylie Webb, speech–language pathologist, where she gives some examples of how she has conducted patient observation outside the clinic (**Video 5.3**).

5.3.4 Patient and Family Self-Report

Patient- and family-centered assessment in speech–language pathology and audiology should typically incorporate patient and family self-report measures. Hence, speech–language pathologists and audiologists should be aware of psychometrically sound self-report questionnaires that can be used to obtain important information about the patients' and families' everyday experiences living with a communication disability. For adults and older children with communication disability, it is important to assess their own perception of their communication functioning; however, at times this self-report can be complemented with "proxy" report, whereby the patient's family reports on the patient's functioning. Of course sometimes, you as the clinician will rely solely on proxy report, particularly when you are working with young children or patients with cognitive difficulties who may not be able to complete self-report measures.

There are a plethora of patient and family self- and proxy-report measures available in audiology and speech–language pathology. In audiology, a systematic review of self-report measures for adult patients with hearing loss identified 39 different standardized questionnaires.[11] It is not the purpose of this chapter to identify specific tools; however, we will mention one commonly used questionnaire for children with hearing loss: the Parent Evaluation of Aural/Oral Performance of Children (PEACH) Scale.[12] Parents are asked to observe their child, and keep a diary of the observations, for example, *"You are in a quiet place with your child. When you ask her a simple question or to do a simple task, does she respond the first time you ask?"* Parents are encouraged to record as many actual instances of this occurring as they can, for example, *"I was sitting quietly with my child and I asked "Where's the book?" and he went and got it."* The clinician and the parents then discuss the observations at the assessment appointment. In acknowledging the broad definition of "family" and the importance of collecting self-report data from others involved in the patient's life, for older children with hearing loss who are in school, there is a similar tool to obtain input from teachers: the Teacher's Evaluation of Aural/oral performance of Children (TEACH).[13] Although these questionnaires are specifically designed for children with hearing loss, the concept of a home diary could be applied to other patients with other communication disorders and their families. Teresa Ching, a researcher in Australia who developed the PEACH and TEACH shares the benefits of using parent self-report as part of a patient- and family-centered approach to assessment (see box on next page "A Word from a Research Expert").

In speech–language pathology, Brandenburg et al[14] identified 29 self-report measures, which evaluate an adult's participation in life activities. The Communicative Participation Item Bank[15–17] provides a very useful list of everyday activities that adults participate in (e.g., talking with people they know, communicating in a small group of people). For each item, patients report if their condition interferes with their communication *not at all, a little, quite a bit, or very much*. Kathryn Yorkston describes the development of the item bank at https://www.youtube.com/watch?v=BrBoB22HLXs. Another common self-report measure used for adult patients in rehabilitation is the Subjective Index of Physical and Social Outcome (SIPSO).[18] The above self- and proxy reports are just a few examples of how you can evaluate a patient and his or her family's biopsychosocial functioning from their perspectives, and we encourage you to seek out other measures.

Of course, in acknowledging the family as the unit of attention in PFCC, there is also a range of self-report measures for families, which enable them to report on the impact of the patient's communication disability on their own functioning, in other words, their third-party disability. Although there are not as many third-party disability self-report measures as patient self-report measures, some commonly used tools for assessing third-party functioning in family members include the Significant Other Scale for Hearing Disability (SOS-HEAR)[19] for spouses of older adults with hearing impairment, and the PedsQL Family Impact Module[20] for parents. These questionnaires can be used in PFCC assessment to provide a

A Word from a Research Expert

Teresa Ching, Audiologist, Australia

The PEACH and TEACH scales[12,13] have been developed for systematic evaluation of auditory/oral performance of children in real-world environments, based on observations of parents and teachers, respectively. They are now used as part of standard clinical protocols for aural rehabilitation of young children with hearing loss in Australia and other parts of the world. By drawing on parents' observations, the scales play a central role in building rapport with parents in family-centered intervention. As a parent puts it,

"It's nice to know what behaviors to observe in daily life following the instructions and questions in the booklet. I especially like those questions including quiet and noisy situation, which help me to pay attention to my child's auditory performance in different environments."

Clinicians introduce the PEACH scale soon after early hearing aid fitting to engage with families and to monitor their child's progress with amplification. The information provided by the PEACH complements other audiologic information to guide ongoing intervention. A clinician from Taiwan indicated that:

"I am giving the PEACH questionnaires to parents at first. As keeping track of their children's auditory behaviors by writing down their performance is also a good training for the parents to learn to be proactive, which is considered an important part in the family-centered early intervention. I then give the PEACH rating scales to those parents with experience using the PEACH questionnaires in the following auditory management. As they are familiar with the questions already, it is intuitive for them to tick the rating scale. Using PEACH or other functional auditory measures is surely complementing other audiological information."

Clinicians have reported that the scales are easy to use and time-efficient in clinical settings. They find that the parents' responses could be used to guide hearing aid fine-tuning, and to support device usage, especially in young children. Reports from clinicians in China suggested that:

"Sometimes the parents of mild to moderate hearing loss kids are reluctant to use hearing aids, and PEACH could give them "evidence" of their kids' performance in real life situations, and that would help them keep using the amplification."

"For severe and profound loss children, PEACH is definitely a good tool to evaluate the auditory performance. This could speed up the cochlear implant (CI) referral."

Recently, the PEACH scale has been updated to include a scale on listening effort, known as the PEACH Plus. The clinical use of the scales has been summarized by a specialist pediatric audiologist:

"The normative data is so important as it gives a valuable benchmark as a comparison with a child's performance and can be used then as a counseling tool to help parents understand where their child is at in comparison to the norm. With preverbal children or children who have no spoken language for other reasons, this is invaluable.

Postoperatively, it is wonderful to be able to plot the progress of the child and discuss with the parents. If the child is not progressing as we would like, it of course is an invaluable tool for looking at where the main difficulties are and to tailor the habitation to those areas."

The PEACH and PEACH Plus, as well as the TEACH and TEACH Plus, are available in multiple languages for use in different countries and free downloads can be found at www.outcomes.nal.gov.au/peach and www.outcomes.nal.gov.au/teach. A self-report version of the PEACH, known as the Self Evaluation of Listening Function (SELF), is also available. Via the same web link, you can view a video demonstration on test administration, and/or get in touch with the researchers who developed the scales.

reliable indication of the effects of a patient's communication disability on family third-party disability and health-related quality of life.

A new approach to individually assessing real-world performance of patients and families, called Ecological Momentary Assessment (EMA), has recently been applied in audiology, and Barbra Timmer, an audiologist in Australia, describes her experience of using this type of patient- and family report (see box on next page "A Word from a Research Expert: Identifying Patient and Family Member Functioning through Ecological Momentary Assessment").

Barbra Timmer, Audiologist, Australia

A commonality across the many available questionnaires that provide measures of self-reported hearing difficulty is that all require input from the individual based on his or her memory and experience of specific listening situations which may, or may not, be important to that individual. Ecological momentary assessment (EMA), or experience sampling, is a data capture technique that involves individuals describing their experiences in real time, in their own natural environment (Shiffman, Stone, and Hufford,[21]). Therefore, with EMA you can find out about a patient's experiences in real time and at multiple times per day, rather than relying on generalized, retrospective self-reports of experiences that may date back several weeks or months.

EMA has been used in various health fields to investigate conditions such as chronic pain, substance addiction, eating disorders, and mental health disability but has had limited use in hearing research. Previous EMA audiology studies have investigated effects of tinnitus, the communication difficulties of individuals with hearing impairment, and the effects of hearing aids with different features.

The EMA technique can incorporate the use of pen-and-paper questionnaires/diaries or mobile devices, the latter having the benefit of triggering or reminding the individual to complete a survey based on particular events or conditions. In some recent research I conducted as part of my PhD studies, I used both time and environmental loudness trigger to ask individuals with hearing impairment to complete a survey. The survey incorporated questions about the listening situation, the acoustic environment, and asked individuals to rate their hearing ability in that situation. The study showed the use of EMA with older adults with mild hearing impairment was feasible and valid, and the technique provided rich data on communication situations and hearing disability.

EMA has also been used in other health sciences to detect intervention effects. In a follow-up EMA study, I assessed 10 of the 29 participants from the first study to investigate if the EMA technique could detect changes in communication performance before, during, and after the provision of hearing aids. Results showed the technique was sufficiently sensitive to detect these changes and concluded that the use of hearing aids does provide benefit to adults with mild hearing impairment. However, individual variation was high, both in terms of amount of benefit, and when hearing aids were helpful. For example, some individuals showed marked benefit from the use of hearing aids in terms of reduced listening effort and others in terms of improved enjoyment of listening situations.

My research using EMA indicated that the technique affords a real-world approach to measuring hearing disability and intervention outcomes. Furthermore, EMA has the potential to provide valuable information to clinicians. A user-friendly EMA app, available to be installed by the individual or his or her clinician on the individual's own smartphone, for example, could facilitate EMA to move from a research to a clinical tool. Data from such an app could be valuable to clinicians to help them determine candidacy for hearing aids and to quantify the benefits of hearing aids for patients who may query their efficacy.

When considering whether to use patient and family self-report measures, it is important to consider the communication accessibility of such measures and whether they would be appropriate for the patient to complete. It is also important to consider the purpose of including the questionnaire, whether or not the content is appropriate for your patients and their families, and how you will incorporate the information in the overall assessment. A limitation of such measures is that they typically use a standard set of items, which may not be appropriate for all patients and families.

5.3.5 Formal Assessment

When conducting a PFCC assessment, it can be tempting to start with a predetermined formal assessment; however, your test selection should instead be guided by concerns identified in the case history and other information obtained through your preassessment planning, patient and family observations, and patient and family self-report. It is also relevant to be mindful that there may be instances where conducting a formal assessment/s is not the most appropriate assessment path for the patient and/or doing so would not be in accordance with patient or family member preferences. It is vital that you be flexible and open to considering whether a comprehensive formal assessment is in the best interest of the patient and family. For example, you should consider the time available for assessment, financial implications for the patient and family, patient and family priorities, previous assessments completed, and what normative data is available for the formal assessments and how this relates to the patient. Speech–language pathologists and audiologists should also consider if commencing "diagnostic therapy" is more appropriate in individual circumstances. This is when the clinician gets underway with trialing an intervention/s and uses the patient's progress to guide decisions regarding further assessment and management. Of course, there will be occasions when completing a formal assessment is paramount for obtaining the information required, for example, to determine the most appropriate communication/listening device, to access services, and to meet funding eligibility requirements which can assist both the patient and his or her family. Thus, the completion of formal assessment/s should be considered according to individual patient and family needs with careful consideration of what information the formal assessment will provide and recognition of why this information is needed at that particular point in time for the patient and his or her family.

Before conducting a patient- and family-centered formal assessment, it is relevant for speech–language pathologists and audiologists to consider (1) how families can be involved in the formal assessment of the patient with the communication difficulty; and (2) if there are formal assessments that the family member could complete, which either provide information about the patient or how the patient's communication difficulty impacts him or her (i.e., third-party disability). Although speech–language pathologists and audiologists need to adhere to standard administration practices when conducting formal assessments, this should not preclude the involvement of family. Crais and colleagues[8] describe ways in which family can be involved during pediatric assessment activities, many of which are also relevant when working with adult patients and their families. Some examples are giving the family choice to be present for all assessment activities;

giving the family a choice to write down observations during the assessment; explaining the purpose of the assessment to the family and ensuring that during the assessment clinicians make comments about what the patient can do well. In addition, Boone and Crais[22] provide several examples of validating questions that clinicians striving for a family-driven assessment can ask family members: *Are we getting a representative sample of what [patient's name] can do?; Was that a correct interpretation of what [patient's name] just said/did?; How could we approach this task in a way that would help [patient's name] feel more comfortable doing it?*

Student Activity 5.6: Triangulating Assessment Data

Consider again the cases of Emily, Shane, and Andrew.

Emily's pure-tone audiogram shows a mild–moderate hearing loss from 250 to 8,000 Hz in both ears; however, her self-report questionnaires indicate more widespread problems. In terms of activities, she has a lot of difficulty understanding speech in the presence of any noise—she manages, but it requires a great deal of effort and makes her very tired. In terms of participation, she reports feelings of embarrassment and self-consciousness in social situations. Work in small groups to discuss how you would talk to Emily and Hugh about these findings.

You reassess Shane's speech and it appears to be the same as it was in the previous assessment 6 months ago. Nevertheless, Lorna reports that she is having increasing difficulty understanding Shane. Work in small groups and brainstorm how you might address these differences in assessment results with Shane and Lorna.

Miranda and Flynn are reporting that Andrew is not responding to their communication attempts at home; however, when you assess him in the clinic, he consistently responds to your attempts to communicate, using a combination of Key Word Sign and single words. Work in small groups to brainstorm how you would discuss these different observations with Miranda and Flynn.

5.3.6 Interdisciplinary Assessment

The information presented in this chapter refers to traditional speech–language pathology and audiology assessments that are typically face-to-face and clinic based conducted by the clinician with patient and family. In Chapter 4, however, we discussed the opportunities for an optimal level of PFCC if an interdisciplinary model of service delivery could be employed. For example, it is most likely that the cases discussed in this book are seen separately by a speech–language pathologist, an audiologist, and a myriad of other health professionals depending on their needs. How much more family centered would it be for them to have at least some level of coordination and integration?

Student Activity 5.7: Interdisciplinary Assessment

Consider again the cases of Emily, Shane, and Andrew and imagine that you work in a setting that includes other professionals, including speech–language pathologists, audiologists, occupational therapists, physiotherapists, and psychologists. Discuss each case and how you could work with these other professionals to address the communication disability experienced by Emily, Shane, Andrew, and their families. After this discussion, consider the benefits of this interdisciplinary perspective for each case and the challenges it might pose for you as a clinician.

5.4 Sharing Assessment Results in a Patient- and Family-Centered Way

Typically, an assessment appointment concludes with a discussion with patients and families about the findings from the assessments and what the next steps will be. As a patient- and family-centered speech–language pathologist and audiologist, you need to consider how you will discuss assessment results with patients and families in a sensitive and respectful way. Gerard William, an audiologist in Australia, who has a hearing loss himself, describes the sensitive nature of providing a diagnosis and explaining assessment results (**Video 5.4**).

Although it may not be possible to provide all of the assessment results immediately after conducting an assessment (since some assessments require further scoring and analysis), it is best practice to provide a verbal summary during the appointment and follow up with a detailed written report and/or make an appointment to verbally report final results. You also need to be mindful that different patients and different family members will likely vary in the level of detail they would like when presenting assessment results. For example, some families will be happy for speech–language pathologists or audiologists to share both positive and negative assessment results, including standard scores, percentile ranks, degrees of severity, and age equivalents. On the other hand, some patients and families may prefer just a short summary of the practical implications of the communication disability. Irrespective of how much "depth" is preferred by the patient and family, as a patient- and family-centered clinician, you should always maintain a strength-based perspective by highlighting what the patient and family can do well, not only what is difficult and challenging for them.

Crais and colleagues[8] have identified 13 family-centered practices for sharing assessment information and results. These include asking patients and families about their feelings/reactions to the assessment results; summarizing conclusions after sharing results with patients and their families; giving choice about when and where the assessment results will be discussed, and spending time identifying the next steps for everyone involved.

Importantly, when summarizing assessment information and potentially providing diagnoses, as a patient- and family-centered clinician, you need to recognize that patients and families are likely to perceive this information as "bad news." In a recent survey, 86% of speech–language pathologists reported that they delivered bad news, and often felt anxious or sad before, during, and after the delivery.[23] Importantly, this can impact the *way* in which you deliver the bad news which can subsequently impact how it's received by the patient and his or her family, and can either lead to confusion and distress or acceptance and healthy adjustment.[24] If you as a clinician regularly describe assessment results and provide diagnoses on a day-to-day basis, you may become blasé about delivering bad news and could be perceived by the patient and family as aggressive in your delivery. On the other hand, if you were anxious or apprehensive about delivering bad news, you could be perceived by the patient and family to be "pussy-footing" around the issue.[23,31] Rebecca Bennett, an audiologist in Australia, shares her experiences in delivering "bad news" to patients and families and provides some practical suggestions for doing this in a sensitive way (see below).

A Word from a Research and Clinical Expert: Use of the SPIKES Model for Breaking Bad news in Speech Pathology and Audiology

Rebecca Bennett, Audiologist, Australia

I once asked a group of 30 experienced audiologists attending a workshop how often they are in the position of breaking bad news to their patients. Most of the clinicians in the room said "never," one of them said "once, when she detected an acoustic neuroma." This group of audiologists had become so comfortable with their role in diagnosing hearing loss that they had forgotten that to the patient, the diagnosis was "bad news."

"Bad news" can describe any information that adversely affects an individual's view of his or her future; whether the news is severe enough to be considered bad is determined by the receiver of the news. The news may be deemed "bad" if it causes a feeling of no hope, a threat to a person's mental or physical well-being, a risk of upsetting an established lifestyle, or where a message is given which conveys to an individual fewer choices in his or her life.[25] As speech–language pathologists and audiologists, we perform and discuss the results of communication and hearing assessments every day. It is important, however, not to lose site of the fact that while it might be our 457th CELF-5 or audiogram, it is often our patient's first. Furthermore, while communication disability may not seem like such a bad prognosis to us, it can have an enormous impact on the patient and family sitting in front of us. Although we assume that patients and/or their families are aware of their communication disability, many may not be fully aware of the severity or the long-term impact of the communication disability. It is not uncommon for patients and families to assume that the communication disability can be easily fixed.

It is also important to consider the personal or psychological impact of the diagnosis. Communication disability represents different things to different people. I will always remember the response from one of my patients when I explained his results to him and confirmed that he did have a significant and permanent hearing loss, he said "Oh no, my wife was right!". He and his wife had spent years debating whether the cause of their communication breakdowns was due to her mumbling or him having a hearing loss. In one foul swoop my diagnosis gave her bragging rights. In all seriousness though, the social stigma associated with communication disability can influence people's perceptions of self when they receive a diagnosis. Unfortunately, societal messages (such as media headlines and advertising) often suggest that communication disability such as hearing impairment is a sign of reduced cognitive function or old age, and that it is a disability that prevents us from achieving our goals. This is not the lived experience of everyone with communication disability and can have a negative impact on a person's inclination to seek help. Similarly, such concepts can affect the way a person understands and reacts to his or her diagnosis.

Before describing the results of the communication or hearing assessment, ask the patient and his or her family how they think the assessment went. Let them consider, explore, and describe their thoughts and feelings regarding their performance first. If they say that they felt they did not do well, then you can let them know that the results agree and then describe the results within the context of how they described their difficulties. However, if the patient indicates that they thought they did well, then a summary of the assessment results and subsequent diagnosis will need to be approached differently, more gently, and perhaps with a conversation surrounding the invisibility of communication disability.

Breaking bad news does not only apply to the diagnosis of communication disability. It can also apply when discussing treatment options. In a similar way to that described above, it can be helpful to ask the patient and family what they expect from the appointment, what treatment options they expect to be discussing. Understanding the patient's and family's expectations regarding treatment options can assist you to tailor the conversation in a way that can be processed by the patient. Use of patient decision making tools (see Chapter 6) can assist with such conversations.

Continued ▶

Despite the fact that speech–language pathologists and audiologists are responsible for delivering bad news, they have been shown to lack both confidence and skill in performing this task.[26] For example, Gilbey[26] conducted a qualitative study to assess parents' experiences with receiving the bad news of the detection of their child's hearing loss; 50% of parents expressed dissatisfaction with the process of breaking of the bad news, specifically the way in which information was imparted bluntly and without empathy.

Breaking bad news is a complex communication task: comprising the verbal component of delivering the news, body language employed when delivering the news, the need to respond to patients' emotional reactions, understanding patients' expectations, involving the patient in decision making, and inclusion of family members. The complexity of the interaction can sometimes create serious miscommunications, such as misunderstanding of the prognosis, treatment options, or treatment regimes.[27–29] Thus, breaking bad news well is an essential skill for all health care professionals. To assist clinicians when disclosing unfavorable information to patients about their health condition, Baile et al[30] developed a six-step protocol called the SPIKES:

- **S = Set up the interview.** Ideally, bad news should be delivered in person and not over the telephone or via a medical report. Ensure that you are in a private, comfortable setting, that the patient has been given the opportunity to bring family members to the appointment, and that you will not be interrupted. Where possible, make sure you are aware of all of the facts relating to the case, that is, read the case notes prior to the appointment, understand the patient's and family's expectations and goals for rehabilitation.
- **P = Assess the patient's and family's perception.** As described earlier, before you begin an explanation, ask the patient and family open-ended questions to find out how they perceive the situation and what they understand or expect regarding treatment options. In this way you can correct any misunderstanding the patient and/or family may have and tailor the news to the patient's and family's understanding and expectations. Terms that are used or avoided, tone of voice, and emotional content of the patient's and family's statements will provide information about their level of understanding and whether the implications of the information have been taken in.
- **I = Obtain the patient's and family's invitation.** Find out how much detail and information the patient and family want regarding their diagnosis and treatment options, as well as the level of technicality with which these conversations should occur.
- **K = Give knowledge and information to the patient and family.** Use language that the patient and family will understand and regularly check in to ensure they understand. Communicate in ways that help the patient and family process the information, for example, use of diagrams or analogies, as well as use of common language and avoidance of technical terms. It can also be beneficial to describe the impact of the hearing loss in ways that match their initial reports of their experiences of the hearing loss or goals for rehabilitation.
- **E = Address the patient's and family's emotions with empathic responses.** Patients' and families' responses can vary from silence to distress, denial, anger, or acceptance. Observe the patient and his or her family and give them time to process the information presented. Allow silence. Allow expression of emotion without criticism. Empathic reflection, identifying the patient's and family's primary emotion and acknowledging their response to the information received, lets them know you have registered what they are conveying to you in words or body language.
- **S = Develop a strategy and a summary.** Summarize the diagnosis and briefly present all treatment options again, being sure to align your information with what you ascertained to be the patient's and family's knowledge, expectations, and hopes. If the patient has his or her family with him or her, allow them time to discuss their thoughts and feelings with each other. You may feel inclined to offer to leave the room while they discuss the assessment results and treatment options you have provided. It is important to reassure the patient and family that there is no rush to decide on treatment and that they may wish to take the information home with them to consider more thoroughly. Be sure not to place pressure on them.

5.5 Summary

In this chapter, we described patient- and family-centered ways to undertake speech–language pathology and audiology assessments including how to engage with patients and families, before, during, and after assessment. Principles discussed in the early chapters of the book are reinforced here with special attention given to the communication skills needed to effectively engage with patients and families at this critical time. Although the focus is on traditional clinician-delivered in-person services, many of the strategies and tips included in this chapter could be applied to other models of service delivery in which assessments are conducted, such as telepractice, mobile and interdisciplinary services (see Chapter 4).

5.6 Reflections

Please respond to the following reflection questions in your PFCC journal:

1. What is the value of a patient and/or family self-report measure in speech–language pathology and audiology? What is one example of such a measure appropriate for patients with communication disorders?

2. What do the letters in the acronym SPIKES stand for in relation to providing assessment results to patients and their families?

3. Consider a recent speech–language pathology or audiology clinical assessment that you participated in. How can you be sure that the information obtained in the clinic is a valid representation of the experiences of the patient in the real world? If you are not sure, what else could you have done to determine this?

References

[1] World Health Organization. ICF, International Classification of Functioning, Disability and Health. Geneva: World Health Organization; 2001

[2] Hebbeler K, Rooney R. Accountability for services for young children with disabilities and the assessment of meaningful outcomes: the role of the speech–language pathologist. Lang Speech Hear Serv Sch. 2009; 40(4):446–456

[3] Hanson SMH. Family health care nursing: An introduction. In: Hanson SMH, Gedaly-Duff V, Kaakinen JR, eds. Family Health Care Nursing: Theory, Practice and Research. 3rd ed. Philadelphia, PA: F. A. Davis; 2005:1–38

[4] Singh G, Hickson L, English K, et al. Family-centered adult audiologic care: a Phonak position statement. Hearing Review. 2016; 23(4):16–21

[5] Crais ER. Working with families of young children with communication and language impairments: intervention and assessment. In: Watts Pappas N, McLeod S, eds. Working with Families in Speech-Language Pathology. San Diego, CA: Plural; 2008:111–130

[6] King GA, Servais M, Bolack L, Shepherd TA, Willoughby C. Development of a measure to assess effective listening and interactive communication skills in the delivery of children's rehabilitation services. Disabil Rehabil. 2012; 34(6):459–469

[7] Kertoy MK, Poulsen AA. Using language to motivate. In: Ziviani J, Poulsen AA, Cuskelly M, eds. The Art and Science of Motivation: A Therapist's Guide to Working with Children. London; Philadelphia, PA: Jessica Kingsley Publishers; 2013:159–191

[8] Crais ER, Roy VP, Free K. Parents' and professionals' perceptions of the implementation of family-centered practices in child assessments. Am J Speech Lang Pathol. 2006; 15(4):365–377

[9] Prelock PA, Beatson J, Bitner B, Broder C, Ducker A. Interdisciplinary assessment of young children with autism spectrum disorder. Lang Speech Hear Serv Sch. 2003; 34(3):194–202

[10] Hersh DLW, O'Halloran R, Brown K, Grohn B, Rodriguez A. Assess for success: evidence for therapeutic assessment. In: Simmons-Mackie N, King J, Beukelman D, eds. Supporting Communication for Adults with Acute and Chronic Aphasia. Baltimore, MD: Paul H Brookes Publishing; 2013:145–164

[11] Granberg S, Dahlström J, Möller C, Kähäri K, Danermark B. The ICF Core Sets for hearing loss—researcher perspective. Part I: systematic review of outcome measures identified in audiological research. Int J Audiol. 2014; 53(2):65–76

[12] Ching TYC, Hill M. The Parents' Evaluation of Aural/Oral Performance of Children (PEACH) scale: normative data. J Am Acad Audiol. 2007; 18(3):220–235

[13] Ching TYC, Hill M, Dillon H. Effect of variations in hearing-aid frequency response on real-life functional performance of children with severe or profound hearing loss. Int J Audiol. 2008; 47(8):461–475

[14] Brandenburg C, Worrall L, Rodriguez A, Bagraith K. Crosswalk of participation self-report measures for aphasia to the ICF: what content is being measured? Disabil Rehabil. 2015; 37 (13):1113–1124

[15] Baylor CR, Yorkston KM, Eadie TL, Miller RM, Amtmann D. Developing the communicative participation item bank: Rasch analysis results from a spasmodic dysphonia sample. J Speech Lang Hear Res. 2009; 52(5):1302–1320

[16] Yorkston KM, Baylor CR, Dietz J, et al. Developing a scale of communicative participation: a cognitive interviewing study. Disabil Rehabil. 2008; 30(6):425–433

[17] Baylor C, Yorkston K, Eadie T, Kim J, Chung H, Amtmann D. The Communicative Participation Item Bank (CPIB): item bank calibration and development of a disorder-generic short form. J Speech Lang Hear Res. 2013; 56(4):1190–1208

[18] Kersten P, George S, Low J, Ashburn A, McLellan L. The Subjective Index of Physical and Social Outcome: its usefulness in a younger stroke population. Int J Rehabil Res. 2004; 27(1):59–63

[19] Scarinci N, Worrall L, Hickson L. The effect of hearing impairment in older people on the spouse: development and psychometric testing of the significant other scale for hearing disability (SOS-HEAR). Int J Audiol. 2009; 48(10):671–683

[20] Varni JW, Sherman SA, Burwinkle TM, Dickinson PE, Dixon P. The PedsQL Family Impact Module: preliminary reliability and validity. Health Qual Life Outcomes. 2004; 2:55

[21] Shiffman S, Stone AA, Hufford MR. Ecological momentary assessment. Annual Review of Clinical Psychology. 2008;4: 1-32.

[22] Boone HA, Crais E. Strategies for achieving family-driven assessment and intervention planning. Young Except Child. 2009; 3(1):2–11

[23] Gold R, Gold A. Delivering bad news: attitudes, feelings, and practice characteristics among speech-language pathologists. Am J Speech Lang Pathol. 2018; 27(1):108–122

[24] Fallowfield L, Jenkins V. Communicating sad, bad, and difficult news in medicine. Lancet. 2004; 363(9405):312–319

[25] Dosanjh S, Barnes J, Bhandari M. Barriers to breaking bad news among medical and surgical residents. Med Educ. 2001; 35(3):197–205

[26] Gilbey P. Qualitative analysis of parents' experience with receiving the news of the detection of their child's hearing loss. Int J Pediatr Otorhinolaryngol. 2010; 74(3):265–270

[27] Gaston CM, Mitchell G. Information giving and decision-making in patients with advanced cancer: a systematic review. Soc Sci Med. 2005; 61(10):2252–2264

[28] Leighl NB, Butow PN, Tattersall MHN. Treatment decision aids in advanced cancer: when the goal is not cure and the answer is not clear. J Clin Oncol. 2004; 22(9):1759–1762

[29] Martin LR, Williams SL, Haskard KB, Dimatteo MR. The challenge of patient adherence. Ther Clin Risk Manag. 2005; 1(3): 189–199

[30] Baile WF, Buckman R, Lenzi R, Glober G, Beale EA, Kudelka AP. SPIKES—a six-step protocol for delivering bad news: application to the patient with cancer. Oncologist. 2000; 5(4): 302–311

[31] Heron J. Helping the Client: A Creative Practical Guide. 5th ed. London: Sage Publications; 2001

Chapter 6

Meeting Patient and Family Member Needs through Collaborative Management Planning

6 Meeting Patient and Family Member Needs through Collaborative Management Planning

Louise Hickson, Carly Meyer, Nerina Scarinci

Abstract

The management of children and adults with communication disability and their families should be a collaborative process from start to finish. This chapter focuses specifically on collaborative goal setting, shared decision making, and the importance of measuring outcomes for patients and their families. In order to make the management process to be truly patient- and family-centered, speech–language pathologists and audiologists must focus on the early establishment of an effective therapeutic relationship. This will ensure that patients and families have trust in the health professional and they feel comfortable when participating in goal setting and decision making processes. In this chapter, a range of tools are described which can help to facilitate collaborative management planning in speech–language pathology and audiology, including shared goal setting approaches, decision aids, reflective communication tools, and outcome measures that evaluate patient and family goals.

Keywords: patient-centered care, family-centered care, management, goal setting, shared decision making, outcome measurement

Learning Objectives

In this chapter, student speech–language pathologists and audiologists will learn the following:

1. Techniques for collaborative goal setting with patients with communication disability and their families.
2. How decision aids can facilitate shared decision making for patients and their families.
3. The importance of measuring outcomes of patient- and family-centered care in speech–language pathology and audiology.

6.1 Introduction to Meeting Patient and Family Member Needs through Collaborative Management Planning

"Shared decision making is seen as a hallmark of good clinical practice, an ethical imperative and as a way of enhancing patient engagement and activation."
(Hoffmann et al, 2014)

Like the assessment process described in Chapter 5, it is important for speech–language pathologists and audiologists to apply the principles of patient- and family-centered care (PFCC) to management planning for patients with communication disability and their families. In this chapter, we will focus specifically on: (1) collaborative goal setting, (2) shared decision making, and (3) measuring outcomes for patients and their families. These three key areas are described initially and, at the end of the chapter, you will be asked to apply the information to the management of the cases featured in this book: Emily and Hugh, Shane and Lorna, and Miranda, Flynn, and Andrew. Before we start talking about collaborative management planning, let's take a moment to think about the patient's perspective and how this should frame goal setting, decision making, and outcome measurement for your speech–language pathology and audiology service. Gerard William, an audiologist in Australia, shares his perspectives on this in **Video 6.1**.

6.2 Collaborative Goal Setting

Once all of the necessary elements of assessment are complete as described in Chapter 5, the next important step is for you to collaborate with the patient and family in order to determine their goals for the treatments that follow. In PFCC, goal setting must focus on the patient and family's biopsychosocial needs, preferences, and context, and importantly, be driven by patients and their families. Although goal setting forms part of the daily practice of speech–language pathologists and audiologists, it can be a foreign concept for patients and families, and therefore the importance of educating patients and families about the goal setting process cannot be underestimated.[1] CanChild, the Centre for Childhood Disability Research, shares some helpful guidelines on how to set collaborative goals with patients and their families, which although was developed for pediatric patients, rings true for adults and children alike: https://www.canchild.ca/system/tenon/assets/attachments/000/001/278/original/FCS13.pdf

In audiology, collaborative goal setting with patients has long been advocated and measures such as the Client Oriented Scale of Improvement

Client Oriented Scale of Improvement

Name : _____ Category : New _____

Audiologist : _____ Return _____

Date : 1. Needs established _____

2. Outcome assessed _____

Specific needs

Indicate order of significance

Degree of change

Final ability (with hearing aid)

Person can hear

10% 25% 50% 75% 95%

	Worse	No difference	Slightly better	Better	Much better	Category	Hardly ever	Occasionally	Half the time	Most of time	Almost always

Categories
1. Conversation with 1 or 2 in quiet
2. Conversation with 1 or 2 in noise
3. Conversation with group in quiet
4. Conversation with group in noise
5. Television/Radio @ normal volume
6. Familiar speaker on phone
7. Unfamiliar speaker on phone
8. Hearing phone ring from another room
9. Hear front door bell or khock
10. Hear traffic
11. Increased social contact
12. Feel embarrassed or stupid
13. Feeling left out
14. Feeling upset or angry
15. Church or meeting
16. Other

Fig. 6.1 Client Oriented Scale of Improvement form for goal setting, prioritizing, and measuring outcomes of hearing aid fitting.

(COSI)[2] (▶ Fig. 6.1) and the Glasgow Hearing Aid Benefit Profile (GHABP)[3] have had widespread adoption. These measures are usually used in the initial assessment appointment after all formal and informal assessments are complete, and they help with the selection of intervention options (e.g., hearing aid fitting, assistive listening device fitting, communication education) that will follow in the next two to three appointments. In speech–language pathology, there are fewer formal tools for collaborative goal setting, although Goal Attainment Scaling (GAS),[4] which is commonly used in rehabilitation settings, has had some application. In Goal Attainment Scaling, the patient and family identify three to four functional goals that they would like to achieve, for example, a goal might be *"for the child to join in two-way conversations with peers, listening and responding to the other side of the conversation."* There is a five-point rating scale and you can specify at the beginning of any treatment what the expected outcomes would be after a certain period of intervention (▶ Fig. 6.2). Typically, in speech–language pathology, you will have a longer-term treatment plan for the patients and their families and you would set both short- (2–3 months) and long-term goals (6–12 months).

In true interprofessional practice, we must also acknowledge the existence of other tools which can be used by interprofessional teams to facilitate patient- and family-centered goal setting. For example, the Canadian Occupational Performance Measure (COPM),[5] which uses a patient- and family-centered approach to identify goals that address important problems in the everyday lives of patients and families across the areas of self-care, productivity, and leisure. What all these goal setting measures and approaches have in common across both speech–language pathology and audiology is the aim of setting SMART goals with patients and their families. The "SMART" acronym was first described in the 1990s and stands for the following:

- **S**pecific—describes the target behavior.
- **M**easurable—quantifies the target behavior.
- **A**ttainable or achievable—target behaviors should be possible for the individual.
- **R**elevant or realistic—target behaviors should be realistic for the individual to undertake.
- **T**ime-limited—target behaviors should be attainable in a certain time frame.

For example, a goal for an adult with hearing loss might be *"I will hear better and join in conversation*

Level of expected outcome after 3 months	Rating	Behavorial statement of expected outcome: Goal 1	Behavorial statement of expected outcome: Goal 2
Much more than expected	+2		
More than expected	+1		
Expected outcome	0		
Less than expected	−1		
Much less than expected	−2		

Fig. 6.2 Goal Attainment Scaling form.

more when I go out to our local restaurant once a week with my husband." Research indicates that more specific and relevant goals lead to the most positive outcomes for patients and families.[6]

Student Activity 6.1: Setting SMART Goals

Work in pairs with another student: one of you is the patient and the other is the clinician. As the patient, think about your health at the moment and consider anything you would like to improve. It could be fitness, weight, stress, sleep patterns, etc. Discuss this with your clinician and develop two SMART goals that relate to what you want to achieve.

Hersh et al[7] investigated goal setting practices with people with aphasia, their family members, and speech–language pathologists and recommended an extended version of SMART goals based on their findings that people with aphasia and their families often felt "confused or excluded" by existing goal setting practices. The frame work is called SMARTER goal setting and provides more guidance regarding the *process* of goal setting than SMART does, which merely specifies the nature of

the final goals. The acronym SMARTER stands for the following:

- **S**hared—sharing the goal setting between patient, family, and clinician.
- **M**onitored—monitoring performance regularly in relation to the goals.
- **A**ccessible—making the goal setting process accessible to the patient with communication disorder.
- **R**elevant—goals should be relevant to the everyday lives of patients and families.
- **T**ransparent—making the link between treatments and achieving goals obvious to all.
- **E**volving—recognizes that goals will change over time.
- **R**elationship-centered—acknowledging that achieving goals depends on relationships between patients, families, and clinicians.

Another interesting and relevant aspect of research conducted by the same team of aphasia specialists[8] was that they mapped the goals identified by people with aphasia during qualitative interviews onto the International Classification of Functioning, Disability, and Health (ICF). The majority of goals people with aphasia talked about were related to activities and participation (e.g., learning to read, speaking, interpersonal interactions, and relationships), although all domains of the ICF were represented. Similarly, in audiology, studies of the goals of adults with hearing impairment have shown that the majority relate to activities and participation (e.g., hearing in noisy situations, listening to TV, joining in social events).[2] When asked about goals, patients and families naturally focus on wanting to achieve things that will help them to function better in the aspects of their daily lives that are most important to them. Clinicians, however, have expert knowledge about the patient's underlying body structure and function changes and for that reason sometimes emphasize impairment goals over activities and participation. An example of an impairment goal would be for a patient to hear more high-frequency sounds. The patient on the other hand would want the goal to be that they could understand more conversation when all the family members are over for dinner. In acknowledging the importance of patient- and family-driven care, any goals you set with patients and families should incorporate both perspectives, and address the patient's and family's biopsychosocial needs, preferences, and context, and should be written in the patient's and family's own words and not the words of the clinician.

As mentioned above, the COSI[2] (▶ Fig. 6.1) is a tool that has been widely adopted in audiology practice to assist with collaborative goal setting between patients and clinicians. When working with the COSI, individual SMART goals are identified and entered as "Specific Needs" on the form. Each goal is then prioritized, with the most important goal being given a "1" in the box provided. Typical goals are categorized on the bottom of the form and often include goals relating to conversation in quiet and in noise, and television and radio listening. Importantly, the COSI can also be used for measuring outcomes, for example, when hearing aids are fitted. After the patient has worn the hearing aids for some weeks, they are asked how much change they have noticed with wearing hearing aids in the situations where they were having difficulties. From the patient's perspective, they are asked to indicate if the goal is worse, no different, slightly better, better, or much better. Patients are also asked how much they can now hear in the particular situation when they wear their hearing aids.

As the COSI is so widely implemented in audiologic practice, sometimes it can be easy for clinicians to lose sight of its purpose and document goals on the COSI only after the patient and his or her family have left the room, or use their own profession-specific language to frame the goals. Obviously when practicing as a PFCC, the COSI should be used collaboratively with patients and families with transparent processes for documenting and evaluating goals. The COSI can also be used to set joint patient–family goals or family-only goals.

The COSI has also been modified for use with adult patients and their family members attending group communication education programs (▶ Fig. 6.3). In

Modified Version of the Client Oriented Scale of Improvement (COSI)

Take a moment to think about what goals you would like to achieve during the group program. Write down your goals in the table below and then number them in the box according to their order of importance.

Name: _____

Date needs established: _____
Date outcome assessed: _____

Specific needs

Indicate order of significance

	Degree of change				
	Worse	No difference	Slightly better	Better	Much better
☐ _____					
☐ _____					
☐ _____					
☐ _____					

Fig. 6.3 Modified version of the Client Oriented Scale of Improvement for goal setting, prioritizing, and measuring outcomes of communication education programs.

Christopher Lind, Audiologist, Australia

On arrival in our clinics, patients and their families often describe their reasons for attending in terms of difficulties in their everyday communication and, by extension, the personal and social consequences. The contexts they report typically involve specific people, and the broader social, physical/acoustic aspects of the environments in which they occur. When discussing these matters with us they make reference not only to the various types of failure in conversation, but the impact on them and their communication partners (CPs), most frequently their family members and close friends.

Everyday talk requires participants in conversation to work cooperatively to establish and maintain shared meaning throughout the conversation. However, there are times when local conversation difficulties occur and typically the people in the conversation work together to address and resolve these. It is with this everyday ability in mind, that family members can be invited into the clinic to discuss the impact of the patient's hearing difficulties and the actions one or other of them might take to overcome them.

Despite the shared responsibility for overcoming these local communication difficulties, case history information in rehabilitative audiology clinical settings is often (a) gathered from the individual with hearing impairment alone, and (b) addresses diagnostic matters at the expense of time spent on the reasons for the individual attending. However, it is these drivers for patients coming to see us in clinic that they wish to have resolved.

The PFCC model is uniquely placed to address patients' presenting complaints in terms of the restrictions they perceive on their participation in everyday interaction as a result of their hearing impairment.

In 2012, the goal-sharing partnership strategy (or GPS) was published which provided an interview strategy to address the presenting communication difficulties, their relative importance, and the methods by which they might best be resolved—as perceived both by the adult with hearing impairment and his or her CP. The GPS (and now the GPS-Mini) grew out of two important events. The first was the development of the Client Oriented Scale of Improvement (COSI), which was a watershed in formalizing and recording assessment of clients' needs and evaluating the outcomes of intervention against these stated everyday needs. The second event was an Ida Institute collaboration that built on the COSI and proposed a new interview method for assessing the *shared* perspectives of the individual with hearing impairment and his/her CP. Involving the CP in goal setting was considered essential since people with hearing impairment and CPs work together in addressing and resolving conversational difficulties in everyday life.

The GPS includes a series of clinical questions that attempt to acknowledge:
- Everyday communication as the most common site of difficulty arising from adult hearing impairment.
- That participants in a conversation share responsibility for its successful conduct and as such the value of acknowledging the perspectives of both the adult with hearing impairment and their CP in identifying the difficulties that arise in everyday communication.
- The situations in which everyday communication is successful, as well as the situations they found communication to be difficult.
- The need to establish shared goals between the patient, the CP, and the clinician to assist in overcoming the perceived communication difficulties.

The GPS-Mini, designed with the time pressures on clinical case history interviews in mind, lays out a series of questions addressed to the patient and the family to assess the everyday conversational difficulties they each/both perceive to be arising. The interview commences with a question to both the adults with hearing impairment and their CP about what (if any) communication go well (e.g., are relaxed, fluent, easy), and what the conditions are that they perceive makes this successful. This allows us a view of the "ideal" or best conditions for our clients. This is followed by asking the patient for the most important situations in which their hearing impairment impacts on communication. Most importantly for each of these, the CPs comment also on their view of the difficulty and the importance of the situation at hand. Following the discussion of these situations offered by the patient, there should be room to ask the CP if there are any additional situations in which they find that their partner's hearing impacts on communication. The

Continued ▶

questioning strategy ends with a conversation about which of these settings is of most importance to the patient and CP to address/resolve.

Typically, this questioning focuses the case history within the context of daily social interaction, and builds a repertoire of social settings in which the hearing impairment limits the patient's ability to "join in." In turn, these situations may be seen as the functional goals against which clinical outcomes might be ultimately measured. ▶ Fig. 6.4 provides a proforma for recording responses to questions using the GPS-Mini.

In summary, the GPS-Mini promotes a family-centered care perspective on needs, goals, intervention, and outcomes. It undoubtedly has application for patients with other communication disorders and could readily be used by speech–language pathologists as well as audiologists.

that instance, outcomes for each goal are measured after the program by asking patients how much change (if any) they have noticed as a result of the program. Hickson et al[9] reported goals set by adults with hearing loss who completed the Active Communication Education (ACE) group program (available for free download at https://shrs.uq.edu.au/active-communication-education-ace). Common goals were: "gain knowledge, and learn communication skills, and develop coping strategies," "learning about specific information, often about hearing aids," and "understanding group conversation." The majority (75%) of 133 participants reported improvements in their first prioritized goal after participating in the ACE program.

More recently, goal setting in audiology appointments has been extended further with the explicit inclusion of family in the process. Preminger and Lind[10] describe the goal-sharing partnership strategy (GPS) and on previous page, Christopher Lind, an audiologist in Australia, describes the latest streamlined version of the GPS.

Although developed in audiology, the COSI and GPS tools could readily be applied to speech–language pathology practice. The collaborative nature of the tools and the commitment to involving patients and families in decisions about interventions are very much in line with recommendations for goal setting for people with other communication disorders such as aphasia. In particular, the Australian Aphasia Rehabilitation Pathway (see http://www.aphasiapathway.com.au/?name=Defining-goal-setting) has been developed as a resource for speech–language pathologists working with patients with aphasia and their families to help them navigate the goal setting process in a patient- and family-centered way.

When working with children with communication disability, the involvement of parents in the goal setting process cannot be underestimated.

Parental involvement has been found to be a key factor in successful outcomes for children with hearing loss,[11] and it is therefore essential that parents (and children as they grow older) are active and valued contributors to any goal setting process. Erbasi et al[12] interviewed parents about how they were involved in the management of their child's hearing loss. A qualitative interview study of a sample of 17 parents was conducted and analysis of the parent interviews found that parents work tirelessly behind the scenes to support their child, act as "case managers," and are always thinking about their child's language development. Unsurprisingly, parents described their role as central to the entire process, and it is therefore important that speech–language pathologists and audiologists acknowledge this in any management planning. As an example of parental involvement, one of the parents in the study described the strategies she had used to reduce background noise at home for her child:

"In designing the house... we knew that this space, having a big open space with lots of glass is always problematic acoustically, so we put the acoustic plasterboard in on the ceiling just to absorb some of the soundwaves so there's not as much reverberation, and also the texture in the ceiling, just not having a plain flat ceiling. We've done things like put the washing machine in a cupboard just to reduce the noise of the washing machine."

Brewer et al[13] review the theories, practical benefits, and challenges of setting collaborative goals with children and their families. Evidence is that setting specific goals is associated with higher levels of performance with intervention and concluded that "the impact of truly collaborative goal setting is sufficiently positive to support organizational and individual time, energy, and resources

GPS-Mini: Developing Shared Goals

"I'd like to get <u>both</u> of your perspectives on the impact hearing loss has on your communication."

Date:	**Person with Hearing Impairment (PHI):**
	Communication Partner (CP):

To both PHI and CP: *When / where do you experience successful communication?*

....

....

To PHI: *What 2 or 3 communication problems do you experience because of your hearing loss?*

    Prompt Question: *How often does this happen?*
    Prompt Question: *What do you do when this happens?*

To CP: *Do you feel that these are problems also?*

Situation 1: ....

PHI's response: ....

CP's reflection / response: ....

Situation 2: ....

PHI's response: ....

CP's reflection / response: ....

Situation 3: ....

PHI's response: ....

CP's reflection / response: ....

To CP: *Are there other communication problem(s) you experience because of your partner's hearing loss? If so, what are they?*
To PHI: *Do you feel that these are problems also?*

Situation: ....

CP's response: ....

PHI's reflection / response: ....

Fig. 6.4 Goal-sharing partnership strategy—Mini for recording shared goals of patients and families.

being invested into making it an integral part of the pediatric rehabilitation process." The authors went on to make recommendations about how to implement collaborative goal setting for children and these were: (1) create a culture that values and supports such goal setting, (2) adopt an explicit goal setting process such as Goal Attainment Scaling, (3) provide support and education for patients, families, and clinicians, and (4) when a number of clinicians are involved, consider appointing a "key worker" who can coordinate goal setting across disciplines.

It can be challenging to engage with young children in goal setting and Missiuna and Pollock[14] describe the Perceived Efficacy and Goal Setting System (PEGS) for use with children aged 5 to 9 years receiving occupational therapy. In their study, children were able to identify fine and gross motor skills they would like to improve with the aid of pictures. You may wish to consider how the PEGS could be adapted for use in speech–language pathology and audiology.

As children grow up, they can participate even more in collaborative goal setting and the Ida Institute describes a very useful tool called "My World" to facilitate this (http://idainstitute.com/toolbox/my_world/). Although designed for children with hearing loss, it would also be applicable to children with other communication disorders. My World is a board game that allows the child to describe his or her day and to think about when he or she has difficulty communicating and when it is easier. A video showing an audiologist using My World with a 7-year-old child can be seen at: http://idainstitute.com/toolbox/my_world/get_started/

The Ida Institute also offers a Transitions Management toolkit to help children with hearing impairment aged 3 to 18 + as they move from childhood to adolescence to adulthood (http://idainstitute.com/toolbox/transitions_management/). It is recommended that clinicians send the link to the toolkit to patients and their families before an appointment and ask them to complete the tools at home and bring them to the appointment.

Student Activity 6.2: Thinking about Goal Setting for Children, Adolescents, and Young Adults

Go to http://idainstitute.com/toolbox/transitions_management/get_started/ and click on one of the five different transition time points for children: 3 to 6 years, 6 to 9 years, 9 to 12 years, 12 to 18 years, or 18 + years.

Undertake the activities for the transition time point you chose: watch the video, read the text, and answer the questions at the bottom of the page based on what you observe in the video. You can save and print out your responses by clicking the Download button.

Now that we've got you thinking about collaborative goal setting with patients and families, and the importance of making these goals SMART, let's hear from Kylie Webb again, a speech–language pathologist in Australia, who shares her tips for working collaboratively with families in early intervention to make your goals and subsequent intervention as practical and functional as possible (**Video 6.2**).

While collaborative goal setting is the most patient- and family-centered way of involving patients and families in setting goals for their intervention program, Kirstine Shrubsole, a speech–language pathologist in Australia, has identified that there are a number of barriers and facilitators to the implementation of collaborative goal setting in clinical practice. Acknowledgement of these potential barriers and facilitators is important if you are to be successful in implementing this approach with your patients and their families.

Kirstine Shrubsole, Speech–Language Pathologist, Australia

As part of a research project, speech–language pathologists were interviewed about their perceived barriers and facilitators to engaging in collaborative goal setting with people with aphasia.[15] Speech–language pathologists working in rehabilitation reported that they engaged in collaborative goal setting with people with aphasia **most of the time** or **always**. Most of these clinicians reported that they dedicated a specific session to goal setting and conducted this in a structured way using specific resources. Several sites had a nominated person within the multidisciplinary team who was responsible for identifying the patient's overall rehabilitation goals, and these were reviewed at weekly case conference meetings ("*Once a week, we review patient goals…you know, where they're at from all disciplines,*" Rehabilitative speech–language pathologist). Speech–language pathologists working in acute or combination roles were more **variable** in their practice, with some clinicians **rarely** engaging in collaborative goal setting. While some reported having their own speech–language pathology goals for the patient, the majority reported many barriers to involving the patient or their family members in this process ("*I guess often patients and family assume the clinician should choose the correct goals. So there's no need for it to be discussed…families don't push for it, neither does the patient.*" Acute speech–language pathologist). The key barriers and facilitators reported by the speech–language pathologists were categorized using the Behavior Change Wheel (described in Chapter 2) as barriers and facilitators relating to Capability (e.g., skills, knowledge, confidence), Opportunity (e.g., physical resources, time), and Motivation (e.g., routine care, belief in benefits)[16] (▶ Fig. 6.5).

Now that you have heard from Kirstine about the potential barriers and facilitators to collaborative goal setting in clinical practice, as a small group, brainstorm possible ways you might be able to address these barriers in a clinical setting, either as a speech–language pathologist or audiologist.

One way you can ensure that your patients and their families are satisfied with their participation in the goal setting process is to ask them if they agree that they had ownership over setting goals, which are meaningful and relevant to them. As health professionals can sometimes struggle getting the balance right in terms of patient, family, and clinician contribution to goal setting, a tool such as the Client-Centeredness of Goal Setting Scale (C-COGS)[17] can be used immediately following the goal setting process.

Importantly, the goal setting process cannot be static. Goals must be regularly reviewed to ensure that they continue to be meaningful and relevant for the patient and family. Therefore, we would like to conclude this section with an example clinical process which can be used to facilitate ongoing patient- and family-centered goal setting. Specifically, the Coaching in Context (CinC) process,[18] which has been used with children with autism spectrum disorder (ASD) and their families, could be applied to any patient with a communication disability and his or her family and is outlined in ▶ Fig. 6.6. The CinC includes a cyclical three-step process beginning with a discussion with the family about what has occurred in the patient's life since the previous intervention session and what progress he or she has made toward achieving his or her goal. Next, the clinician and family brainstorm together what strategies could be used to help achieve their goal. Finally, the family works with the clinician to develop an action plan by selecting, prioritizing, and refining the strategies identified in the brainstorming phase. A key feature of finalizing this process is the documentation of the action plan in writing and the provision of this to the family.[18]

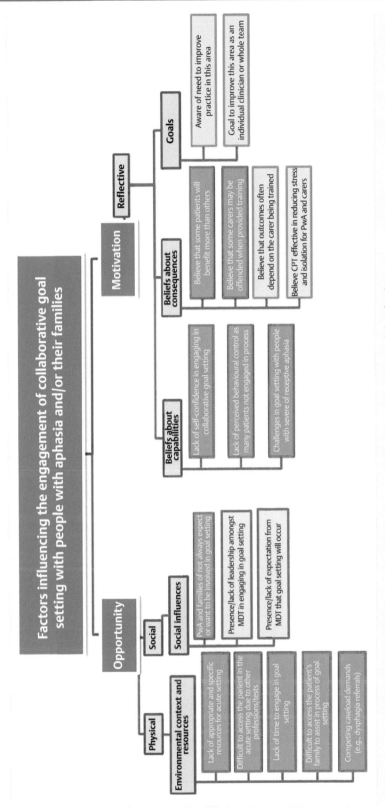

Fig. 6.5 Barriers and facilitators to implementing collaborative goal setting with patients with aphasia and their families.

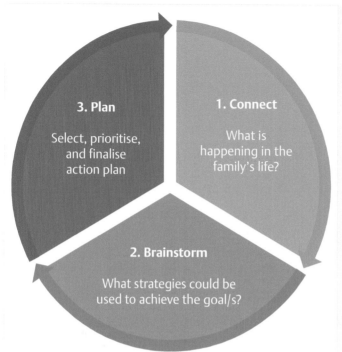

Fig. 6.6 The Coaching in Context (CinC) process.[18]

6.3 Shared Decision Making

When practicing as a patient- and family-centered clinician, after you spend time setting collaborative goals with patients and families, the next logical step is shared decision making where clinicians and patients work together to decide on the best course of action. Shared decision making is a central tenet of PFCC as well-informed decisions are more likely to meet the biopsychosocial needs, preferences, and contexts of patients and their families. In a speech–language pathology and audiology context, these decisions will relate to issues as diverse as the type of intervention approach used to what specialized equipment the patient will need, right through to decisions about the mode and frequency of intervention. Tuchman[19] talks about shared decision making involving two steps. First, decisions must be made about which issues should be prioritized in management, and secondly, which strategies should be implemented to address these priority issues.

Student Activity 6.4: Shared Decision Making in Medicine

Go to the Patient Revolution website: https://patientrevolution.org/ Their mission is to empower patients, families, community advocates, clinicians, and more to rebuild our health care system one bit at a time. Watch the inspiring YouTube video interview of Mayo Clinic Professor of Medicine, Victor Montori, describing shared decision making: https://www.youtube.com/watch?v=NECp7TtEzM4

Discuss these questions:

Dr Montori says the patient, not the health professional, is the "expert." Is that how you think about your patients?

Dr Montori comments on the extra time it takes for shared decision making. On average, it extends consultations by about 10% (2–3 minutes for a 20-minute consultation). What does he say about the "value" of spending that time? What do you think about the possible values of shared decision making?

Dr Montori finishes by inviting you to be part of this "patient revolution" of shared decision making. Do you think he is right? Doesn't this happen all the time now anyway?

Shared decision making has received an enormous amount of attention in health care in developed countries over the last 10 years and this coincides with the rapid expansion of health care information readily available to patients and their families via the internet. Rose et al[20] conducted a systematic review of literature about shared decision making in adult rehabilitation settings. Their findings can be summarized as follows:

- Although shared decision making was encouraged in different settings, it still tended to be the clinician who led the decision making process.
- Clinicians reported the benefits of shared decision making; however, they were concerned that it took too much time.
- Patients reported the benefits of shared decision making although they found it challenging at times because they felt they did not have enough knowledge to make some decisions.
- Both clinicians and patients felt that patients' motivation was higher when they were involved in decisions.
- Shared decision making was facilitated with the use of decision aids that provided information in a structured way.

Another systematic review considered the more recent application of shared decision making in pediatric settings. Wyatt et al[21] identified that shared decision making is an "emerging trend" in pediatric health care with 54 interventions described in the literature. They reported that the majority of interventions engage parents rather than children, and there is limited rigorous research about the impact of shared decision making on outcomes for children. There is some evidence that shared decision making in pediatrics is associated with improved knowledge and reduced decisional conflict.

 Decision aids are tools that can be used to facilitate shared decision making. There are a number of freely available resources, which can help you develop your own decision aids (e.g., the Ottawa Hospital Research Institute Patient Decision Aids https://decisionaid.ohri.ca/). In recent years, the use of decision aids in audiology has received some specific attention, and on next page, Ariane Laplante-Lévesque, an audiologist in Denmark, and Helen Pryce, an audiologist in the United Kingdom, share their experiences using decision aids in audiology.

 As to who should be responsible for making the final decision, in being a truly patient- and family-centered clinician, it is your responsibility to ensure that patients and their families drive their own care, and hence are the ultimate decision makers. As a speech–language pathologist or audiologist, however, you have a key role in facilitating this decision making process by providing information about the patient's functioning and assessment results (Chapter 5), as well as making use of decision aids to highlight the possible intervention options for the patient and family.

 Although shared decision making is considered the best practice in health care especially for patients with chronic health conditions, the evidence suggests that it does not always happen in reality. Krupat et al[27] developed the Four Habits Coding Scheme (4HCS) to help identify effective clinical communication that will allow shared decision making to occur:

Habit 1: Invest in the beginning—show familiarity, greet warmly, engage in small talk, question style, expansion of concerns, elicit full agenda.
Habit 2: Elicit the patient's and family's perspective—patient's and family's understanding of the problem, goals for visit, impact on life.
Habit 3: Demonstrate empathy—encourage emotional expression, accept feelings, identify feelings, show good nonverbal behavior.
Habit 4: Invest in the end—use patient's and family's frame of reference, allow time to absorb, give clear explanations, offer rationale for tests, test for comprehension, involve in decisions, explore plan acceptability, explore barriers, encourage questions, plan for follow-up.

The 4HCS has 23 items and each is scored on a five-point scale with higher scores indicating more effective communication. Krupat et al[27] scored 100 videotaped appointments between 50 physicians and patients in a hospital setting. Results showed that there was a great deal of variability across physicians and that highest mean scores were evident for demonstrating familiarity with the patient, encouraging patients to expand on their concerns, showing appropriate nonverbal behaviors, and avoiding jargon. Lowest scores, and therefore the least effective communication was evident for engaging in small talk, showing interest in the patient's perspective, identifying and accepting patient's emotions, testing for comprehension, and exploring barriers to implementation.

 Another very useful tool to examine clinical encounters is called OPTION (Observing Patient Involvement in Decision Making) developed by

Ariane Laplante-Lévesque, Audiologist, Denmark, and Helen Pryce, Audiologist, United Kingdom

It is challenging for clinicians to bring evidence-based treatment options into clinical practice. Research evidence is often presented as clinical practice guidelines without specific guidance on how to translate what works at a population level to support a specific patient and his or her family at a specific point in time. This is where decision aids come in. They fill the gap between research evidence and your next patient.

Decision aids are "evidence-based tools designed to help patients make specific and deliberated choices among healthcare options"[22](p.7). Decision aids help, rather than replace, the clinician. There is good evidence within general health care that decision aids help people make decisions. A recent Cochrane review of 105 studies noted that there is high-quality evidence of decision aids improving knowledge of options available. There is also high-quality evidence that patients who use decision aids are better informed about what is most important to them. It is also likely that patients develop more accurate expectations about benefits and harms of options and that they participate more in decision making (moderate-quality evidence). It is likely that people who use decision aids make decisions that are in line with their values and preferences. This may lead to greater alignment between clinicians and their patients' and families' preferences.[22]

Within audiology, decision aids have been developed for children undergoing cochlear implantation[23] and for adults with hearing loss.[24] More recently, the Hearing Loss Option Grid (www.optiongrid.org/hearing) and the first decision aid for tinnitus from the British Tinnitus Association were developed. These decision aids were produced through a systematic process of literature review to determine options and research to establish important frequently asked questions about hearing loss and tinnitus. The process of development included multiple iterative stages with focus groups of patients, clinicians, research experts in the field, and experts in decision aids contributing to the refinement of the tools.[25] Both the Hearing Loss Option Grid and the tinnitus decision aid were then refined through user testing and readability testing.

Elwyn and colleagues[26] led a group that devised an international standard system for decision aids. This forms a checklist with items assessing eight domains (information, probabilities, values, decision guidance, development, evidence, disclosure, and plain language) with a further two domains for screening and test decision aids (test and decision screening test information). Key factors in interpreting quality of decision aids are the potential conflicts of interest of those developing them and the reliability of information presented. There are many decision aids for hearing-related issues such as hearing loss options, cochlear implants, and tinnitus. It is better to use a decision aid that has been through a rigorous development process. Look for a decision aid that achieves these four goals:

1. Informs without overloading.
2. Elicits values and preferences.
3. Invites family members to participate in the decision.
4. Prevents decisional conflict/stress.

In summary, we can be confident that decision aids help. There are reliable standards for assessing decision aids and decision aids that pass those standards are available for a number of hearing-related conditions including hearing loss, tinnitus, and cochlear implantation. Therefore, the natural next step is for decision aids to form part of routine clinical practice. The British Tinnitus Association developed a series of short films to demonstrate how you can use the tinnitus decision aid to include patient preferences in the discussion (https://www.youtube.com/watch?v=6726cCoRDrE). Check this video for great tips to enable shared decision making.

Ariane and Helen's Top Tips for Using Decision Aids with Patients with Communication Disability and their Families

Remember, small changes to your everyday practice will come a long way to enabling shared decision making with your patients and their families:

- Ask open questions to explore the perspective of patients and their families regarding intervention options. For example, instead of asking *"Have you thought of hearing aids?,"* ask patients and their families *"What do you think of hearing aids?"*

Continued ▶

- Say explicitly to your patients that you are working alongside them to make the best choices together.
- Not all patients want to be involved in the same way in decisions concerning their care. Offer patients to be involved in every step of decision making, observe their reactions, and adjust accordingly. Think patient- and family-centered!
- Remember that decision aids alone do not guarantee shared decision making. They are a tool to enable good conversations with your patients. Up to you to make the most of them and make shared decisions a reality!

Elwyn and colleagues.[28] Details about the tool along with free downloads of translations into a range of languages can be found at http://www.glynelwyn.com/observer-option-12-2005-2013.html. Twelve behaviors associated with shared decision making make up the items in the OPTION and, for each item, a score from 0 (the behavior is not observed) to 4 (the behavior is observed and executed to a high standard) is given. When the researchers applied the scale to 186 medical consultations, they found that for almost all behaviors, the most frequent score was 0, indicating that shared decision making behaviors were rarely observed. Two behaviors had slightly higher scores (but still 2 or less) and these were: *"The clinician checks that the patient has understood the information"* and *"The clinician offers the patient explicit opportunities to ask questions during the decision making process."*

Student Activity 6.5: Using the OPTION in Clinical Settings to Maximize Shared Decision Making

The OPTION is a checklist that you can use in clinic to either note your observations of other clinicians or to reflect on your own patient interactions. You could use it while you observe another student or a clinician. You could also complete it about your own interaction with a patient and his or her family. Reflect on an appointment you have just completed or watch a video of your appointment and complete the checklist.

It is common for health professionals to get very low scores on the OPTION. What was your average score? On which items were your scores lowest? On which items were your scores highest?

Finish by making a list of ways you could have involved the patient (and his or her family) more in the decision making process. Remember the aim is for "sharing"!

The research presented thus far about the reality of shared decision making in clinical appointments has come from medicine; however, similar low levels of patient and family involvement have also been observed in audiology. Grenness et al[29] analyzed 62 videotaped appointments with adult patients (and family members) attending an audiology clinic for an initial assessment appointment. The interactions were characterized as clinician-centered, rather than patient- or family-centered; the audiologists did the majority of the talking and they presented very limited treatment options (hearing aids only option in 83% of consultations where the patient had a measured hearing impairment). Looking at the same videos, Ekberg et al[30] examined the involvement of families in decision making; for 17 of the 62 appointments a family member accompanied the patient. Overall, family members were typically not invited to join the conversation during the appointment and participated in just 12% of the total talk time during the appointments. It was clear, however, that family members were keen to participate and wanted to share their experiences of the patient's hearing impairment. In summary, the findings suggest that current audiology practice may be a long way from being truly patient- and family-centered and we need to develop communication skills that will allow PFCC to happen.

As you develop your communication skills for collaborative management planning, you may find that you are naturally going to elicit more information about your patients' and families' psychosocial and psychological functioning than you would if you were using a clinician-centered approach to care. Given that our patients have a communication disability, you, as a speech–language pathologist or audiologist, have an important role in supporting patients and families to seek help from a mental health professional when required. On next page, Brooke Ryan, a speech–language pathologist and Ian Kneebone, a clinical psychologist, describe a new approach to psychological care for patients with aphasia and their families called Stepped Psychological Care.

A Word from Two Research Experts: The Role of Stroke Professionals within Stepped Psychological Care for People with Aphasia and Their Families

Brooke Ryan, Speech–Language Pathologist and Ian Kneebone, Clinical Psychologist, Australia

A large proportion of stroke survivors are diagnosed with a mental health condition, and this is particularly true of patients who also have aphasia. Patients with poststroke aphasia report a range of psychological impacts, including changes in identity and sense of self, feelings of frustration and/or isolation, negative self-esteem, reduced coping abilities, stress, distress, reduced optimism and hope, and changed life satisfaction, and well-being.[31–35] Not surprisingly then, up to 70% of patients with stroke and aphasia have depression[36] and up to 40% have anxiety.[37] Family members of patients with aphasia are also prone to developing depression and experience a variety of psychosocial consequences after the onset of aphasia.[38] It is important that speech–language pathologists are aware of the psychological changes that can occur poststroke in patients with aphasia and their families as they are in an ideal position to facilitate access to mental health services when required.

One approach used to manage emotional difficulties and psychological changes poststroke is "stepped psychological care." Kneebone[39] has provided a narrative review and proposed a model for stepped psychological care after stroke. In Kneebone's[39] approach, four levels of intervention are described. Treatments progress from "low-intensity" to "high-intensity" interventions through successive steps. People with stroke enter the stepped care system and have their service level aligned to their requirements and if at any point their condition deteriorates, or if they do not respond to the intervention, they proceed to the next step in the model where the service becomes increasingly tailored, and is delivered by more specialized practitioners. Similarly, someone who has benefitted from a higher-level intervention initially might "step down" and maintain his or her treatment outcome with a less intensive intervention. Compared with stepped care for mental health in other settings, within stepped psychological care after stroke, step one is promoted as being applicable to all. The provision of services such as support groups is seen as preventative and as enhancing psychological well-being. The four intervention levels of Kneebone's[39] stepped psychological care for stroke model include the following:

- Step one interventions that are appropriate for all stroke survivors and for the treatment of "subthreshold problems" such as general difficulties with coping and experiences of general distress.
- Step two interventions that target mild–moderate symptoms of impaired mood.
- Step three interventions that address severe and persistent disorders.
- Step four interventions that address severe challenging behavior.

For more information on the interventions that may be provided at each level of stepped psychological after stroke refer to Kneebone.[39] The delivery of psychological care to people with aphasia and their families is unique because of the very fact that the patient has a communication disability. In ▶ Fig. 6.7, we outline the possible role of a speech–language pathologist within a stepped psychological care after stroke model for patients with aphasia and their families.

6.4 Measuring Outcomes for Patients and Families

Once goals and treatment approaches are agreed on between patients, families, and clinicians, and you have implemented the chosen interventions for patients and their families, it is important to measure the outcomes of the management process. This is where your collaborative goal setting really comes to fruition because if you have set SMART goals with your patients and their families, then you can measure outcomes to determine if these goals have been reached.

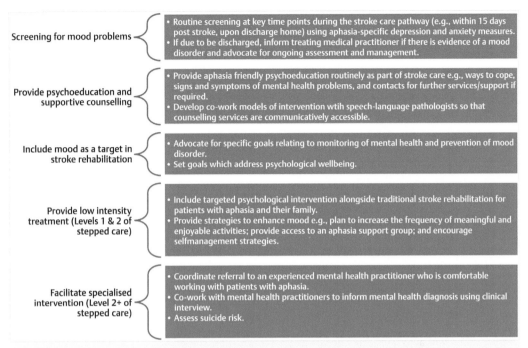

Fig. 6.7 Proposed model of stepped psychological care for patients with aphasia and their families.

Why Measure Patient and Family Outcomes?

- Outcome measures provide evidence for the patients, their families, the clinician, other professionals involved in the patient's care, and those who fund the treatment about the results of the interventions.
- The fact that you are prepared to measure outcomes and not just assume that everything you do benefits the patients and their families demonstrates your commitment to evidence-based practice and to quality improvement.
- If you don't measure outcomes, then others will! This is particularly true if services are being paid for by third-party payers such as insurance companies. They want to know that their members receive value for money.

There are hundreds of outcome measures that have been developed for use in speech–language pathology and audiology and they typically have a number of common features. First, outcome measures are commonly self-report survey measures with the outcome of treatment determined by the patient or, in the case of children, by their parents. A much smaller number of measures exist for family members of adult patients. As discussed in Chapter 5, an example of an audiology outcome measure for families of adults with hearing loss is the Significant Other Scale for Hearing Disability (SOS-HEAR[40]) and an example of a speech pathology measure for families is the PedsQL Family Impact Module.[41] Second, outcomes measures provide information about the individual patient and/or family response to treatment, but the results can also be collated to provide information about the outcomes of a whole service. For example, in audiology, Hickson et al[42] report on the outcomes of a national hearing rehabilitation service in Australia and, in speech–language pathology, Wallace et al[43] report on an international project developing a core set of outcomes measurement for people with aphasia.

Outcomes are also most often measured in relation to the original goals set by the patient and family. When measuring outcomes against goals, the patient and his or her family are asked if goals have been met, partially met, or not met. Many of the goal setting measures, such as the COSI (► Fig. 6.1) and the GAS (► Fig. 6.2) have an outcome measurement component. The clinician, the patient, and the family should discuss the outcomes and reach consensus.

Satisfaction with care is commonly included in outcomes measurement. CanChild at McMaster University in Canada have developed a number of self-report tools called the Measures of Processes of Care (MPOC) that particularly focus on measuring the family-centeredness of health care services. There is a version for parents, a version for adult patients, and a version for service providers https://canchild.ca/. CanChild have developed a very helpful summary of the available MPOC measures, which can be adapted for clinicians to use as checklists to measure the family-centeredness of their service. This information sheet can be downloaded at https://www.canchild.ca/system/tenon/assets/attachments/000/001/283/original/FCS18.pdf

Outcome measurement usually occurs immediately postintervention or a few months afterward. In the case of patients and their families who are receiving ongoing intervention over a long period of time, outcome measurement can occur every 6 months. As speech–language pathologists and audiologists, you are likely to need to modify your management plan in collaboration with patients and their families after outcomes are measured. For example, a patient fitted with a hearing aid might report that he or she is doing better in relation to some goals set initially (e.g., listening to television at a normal volume) but doing less well for other goals (e.g., understanding conversation with three or more people). This suggests that they would likely benefit from further assistance in the form of communication education or possibly an assistive listening device connected to their hearing aids. Similarly, in speech–language pathology, patients and their families may report that they are functioning well in certain communicative environments; however, report more functional difficulties in certain settings, which may require the reevaluation of patient goals, and subsequently, an additional decision making process about future interventions.

Student Activity 6.6: Case Studies of Collaborative Goal Setting and Shared Decision Making

Return to the case studies we have discussed throughout the book: Emily and Hugh, Shane and Lorna, and Miranda, Flynn, and Andrew.

For each case, describe three goals that the patient and family are likely to want to achieve in the next year. Also describe how you would develop the goals, how you would present them to the patient and family members, and how you would measure whether or not the goals had been achieved.

6.5 Summary

Your management of children and adults with communication disability and their families should be a process of collaboration from start to finish. As a speech–language pathologist or audiologist, you are building a therapeutic relationship that is typically long term rather than short term, and the evidence is that the results your patients and families will achieve will be far better if you agree on the treatment plan together from the start and at every step along the way. Treatment is not something done to patients. It is a shared activity of clinicians, patients, and families. There are a number of tools described in this chapter to help you achieve collaborative management planning: shared goal setting approaches, decision aids, reflective communication tools, and outcome measures that evaluate the agreed goals.

6.6 Reflections

Please respond to the following reflection questions in your PFCC journal:
1. What does the acronym SMARTER refer to in relation to setting goals with patients and their families?
2. What are the four key goals of using decision aids in speech–language pathology or audiology practice?

3. Consider a recent speech–language pathology or audiology clinical session you participated in where the patient had to make a decision about further treatment at the end of the session. How was the decision making process structured? Who was involved? Could it have been more "shared" and, if so, how?

References

[1] Leach E, Cornwell P, Fleming J, Haines T. Patient centered goal-setting in a subacute rehabilitation setting. Disabil Rehabil. 2010; 32(2):159–172

[2] Dillon H, James A, Ginis J. Client Oriented Scale of Improvement (COSI) and its relationship to several other measures of benefit and satisfaction provided by hearing aids. J Am Acad Audiol. 1997; 8(1):27–43

[3] Gatehouse S. Glasgow Hearing Aid Benefit Profile: derivation and validation of a client-centered outcome measure for hearing aid services. J Am Acad Audiol. 1999; 10:80–103

[4] McKenna L. Goal planning in audiological rehabilitation. Br J Audiol. 1987; 21(1):5-11

[5] Law M, Baptiste S, Carswell A, McColl MA, Polatajko H, Pollock N. Canadian Occupational Performance Measure. Toronto: CAOT Publications ACE; 1998

[6] Ponte-Allan M, Giles GM. Goal setting and functional outcomes in rehabilitation. Am J Occup Ther. 1999; 53(6):646–649

[7] Hersh D, Worrall L, Howe T, Sherratt S, Davidson B. SMARTER goal setting in aphasia rehabilitation. Aphasiology. 2012; 26 (2):220–233

[8] Worrall L, Sherratt S, Rogers P, et al. What people with aphasia want: their goals according to the ICF. Aphasiology. 2011; 25(3):309–322

[9] Hickson L, Worrall L, Scarinci N. Active Communication Education (ACE): a program for older people with hearing impairment. London: Speechmark; 2007

[10] Preminger JE, Lind C. Assisting communication partners in the setting of treatment goals: The development of the goal sharing for partners strategy. Semin Hear. 2012; 33(1):53–64

[11] Erbasi E, Hickson L, Scarinci N. Communication outcomes of children with hearing loss enrolled in programs implementing different educational approaches: a systematic review. Speech Lang Hearing. 2017; 20(2):102–121

[12] Erbasi E, Scarinci N, Hickson L, Ching TYC. Parental involvement in the care and intervention of children with hearing loss. Int J Audiol. 2018; 57(suppl 2):S15–S26

[13] Brewer K, Pollock N, Wright FV. Addressing the challenges of collaborative goal setting with children and their families. Phys Occup Ther Pediatr. 2014; 34(2):138–152

[14] Missiuna C, Pollock N. Perceived efficacy and goal setting in young children. Can J Occup Ther. 2000; 67(2):101–109

[15] Shrubsole K, Worrall L, Power E, O'Connor D. Understanding practice: factors influencing speech pathologist's adherence to clinical practice guideline recommendations in post-stroke aphasia. In preparation

[16] Michie S, Miles J, Weinman J. Patient-centredness in chronic illness: what is it and does it matter? Patient Educ Couns. 2003; 51(3):197–206

[17] Doig E, Prescott S, Fleming J, Cornwell P, Kuipers P. Development and construct validation of the Client-Centredness of Goal Setting (C-COGS) scale. Scand J Occup Ther. 2015; 22(4):302–310

[18] Potvin MC, Prelock PA, Savard L. Supporting children with autism and their families: a culturally responsive family-driven interprofessional process. Pediatr Clin North Am. 2018; 65 (1):47–57

[19] Tuchman LI. Team dynamics and communication. In: Rosin P, Whitehead A, Tuchman L, Jesien G, Begun A, Irwin L, eds. Partnerships in Family-Centered Care: A Guide to Collaborative Early Intervention. Baltimore: Paul H. Brooks; 1996:145–185

[20] Rose A, Rosewilliam S, Soundy A. Shared decision making within goal setting in rehabilitation settings: a systematic review. Patient Educ Couns. 2017; 100(1):65–75

[21] Wyatt KD, List B, Brinkman WB, et al. Shared decision making in pediatrics: a systematic review and meta-analysis. Acad Pediatr. 2015; 15(6):573–583

[22] Stacey D, Legare F, Lewis K, et al. Decision aids for people facing health treatment or screening decisions. Cochrane Database Syst Rev. 2017; 4:CD001431

[23] Johnston JC, Durieux-Smith A, O'Connor A, Benzies K, Fitzpatrick E, Angus D. The development and piloting of a decision aid for parents considering sequential bilateral cochlear implantation for their child with hearing loss. Volta Review. 2009; 109(2–3):124–141

[24] Laplante-Lévesque A, Hickson L, Worrall L. Factors influencing rehabilitation decisions of adults with acquired hearing impairment. Int J Audiol. 2010; 49(7):497–507

[25] Pryce H, Hall A, Laplante-Lévesque A, Clark E. A qualitative investigation of decision making during help-seeking for adult hearing loss. Int J Audiol. 2016; 55(11):658–665

[26] Elwyn G, O'Connor AM, Bennett C, et al. Assessing the quality of decision support technologies using the International Patient Decision Aid Standards instrument (IPDASi). PLoS One. 2009; 4(3):e4705

[27] Krupat E, Frankel R, Stein T, Irish J. The Four Habits Coding Scheme: validation of an instrument to assess clinicians' communication behavior. Patient Educ Couns. 2006; 62(1):38–45

[28] Elwyn G, Hutchings H, Edwards A, et al. The OPTION scale: measuring the extent that clinicians involve patients in decision-making tasks. Health Expect. 2005; 8 (1):34–42

[29] Grenness C, Hickson L, Laplante-Lévesque A, Meyer C, Davidson B. The nature of communication throughout diagnosis and management planning in initial audiologic rehabilitation consultations. J Am Acad Audiol. 2015; 26(1):36–50

[30] Ekberg K, Meyer C, Scarinci N, Grenness C, Hickson L. Family member involvement in audiology appointments with older people with hearing impairment. Int J Audiol. 2015; 54(2):70–76

[31] Brumfitt S. Psychosocial aspects of aphasia: speech and language therapists' views on professional practice. Disabil Rehabil. 2006; 28(8):523–534

[32] Cruice M, Hill R, Worrall L, Hickson L. Conceptualising quality of life for older people with aphasia. Aphasiology. 2010; 24 (3):327–347

[33] Hilari K, Needle JJ, Harrison KL. What are the important factors in health-related quality of life for people with aphasia? A systematic review. Arch Phys Med Rehabil. 2012; 93(1) Suppl:S86–S95

[34] Parr S. Psychosocial aspects of aphasia: whose perspectives? Folia Phoniatr Logop. 2001; 53(5):266–288

[35] Shadden B, Hagstrom F, Koski P. Neurogenic Communication Disorders. Life Stories and the Narrative Self. San Diego, CA: Plural Publishing; 2008

[36] Kauhanen ML, Korpelainen JT, Hiltunen P, et al. Aphasia, depression, and non-verbal cognitive impairment in ischaemic stroke. Cerebrovasc Dis. 2000; 10(6):455–461

[37] Morris R, Eccles A, Ryan B, Kneebone II. Prevalence of anxiety in people with aphasia after stroke. Aphasiology. 2017; 31 (12):1410–1415

[38] Grawburg M, Howe T, Worrall L, Scarinci N. Third-party disability in family members of people with aphasia: a systematic review. Disabil Rehabil. 2013; 35(16):1324–1341

[39] Kneebone II. Stepped psychological care after stroke. Disabil Rehabil. 2016; 38(18):1836–1843

[40] Scarinci N, Worrall L, Hickson L. The effect of hearing impairment in older people on the spouse: development and psychometric testing of the significant other scale for hearing disability (SOS-HEAR). Int J Audiol. 2009; 48(10): 671–683

[41] Varni JW, Sherman SA, Burwinkle TM, Dickinson PE, Dixon P. The PedsQL Family Impact Module: preliminary reliability and validity. Health Qual Life Outcomes. 2004; 2:55

[42] Hickson L, Clutterbuck S, Khan A. Factors associated with hearing aid fitting outcomes on the IOI-HA. Int J Audiol. 2010; 49(8):586–595

[43] Wallace SJ, Worrall L, Rose T, Le Dorze G. Core Outcomes in Aphasia Treatment Research: An e-Delphi Consensus Study of International Aphasia Researchers. Am J Speech Lang Pathol. 2016; 25 4S:S729–S742

Chapter 7

Consideration of Cultural and Linguistic Diversity in Patient- and Family-Centered Care

7 Consideration of Cultural and Linguistic Diversity in Patient- and Family-Centered Care

Nerina Scarinci, Carly Meyer, Leanne Sorbello

Abstract

Our modern societies are as culturally and linguistically diverse as ever, and this is reflected in the caseloads of speech–language pathologists and audiologists all over the world. This diversity is likely to be seen in all workplace settings. Interestingly, the same level of diversity is not typically observed within health professionals themselves. This has implications for providing culturally and linguistically responsive care. The principles of patient- and family-centered care and culturally and linguistically responsive care are similar, particularly in regard to the provision of individualized and patient- and family-driven care. Like patient- and family-centered care, the provision of culturally and linguistically responsive care has also been found to result in improved outcomes for patients and families.

This chapter will discuss how to be a culturally and linguistically responsive clinician, how to conduct a culturally and linguistically responsive assessment, and lastly, how to implement culturally and linguistically responsive approaches to collaborative management planning.

Keywords: patient-centered care, family-centered care, cultural and linguistic diversity, assessment, management

Learning Objectives

In this chapter, student speech–language pathologists and audiologists will learn the following:

1. Special considerations for being a culturally and linguistically responsive clinician.
2. How to conduct a culturally and linguistically responsive speech–language pathology or audiology assessment with culturally and linguistically diverse (CALD) patients and families?
3. How to engage CALD patients and families in collaborative management planning, including goal setting and decision making?

7.1 Introduction to Cultural and Linguistic Diversity in Patient- and Family-Centered Care

Our modern societies are as culturally and linguistically diverse (CALD) as ever, and this is reflected in the caseloads of speech–language pathologists and audiologists all over the world. This is likely to be the case, irrespective of whether or not you are working in a hospital, private practice, community, or educational setting. Interestingly, the same level of diversity is not typically observed within health professionals themselves. This has implications for providing culturally and linguistically responsive care.[1] By way of example, the first two authors of this chapter, Nerina and Carly, identify themselves as Anglo-Australians who are monolingual Australian English speakers, and the third author, Leanne, is an Italian Australian. Therefore, throughout this chapter, we have invited contributions from other speech–language pathologists and audiologists from a variety of cultural and linguistic backgrounds.

Before we begin, however, we must acknowledge that the principles of patient- and family-centered care (PFCC) and culturally and linguistically responsive care are similar, particularly in regard to the provision of individualized and patient- and family-driven care.[2] Furthermore, just like PFCC has well-documented benefits for patients, families, and clinicians, the provision of culturally and linguistically responsive care has also been found to result in improved outcomes for patients and families, including reduced family stress, improved accessibility to services, and enhanced satisfaction with care.[3] Therefore, many of the concepts and strategies discussed previously in this book will also be applied while working with patients and families from CALD backgrounds. What we discuss in this chapter is intended to extend and challenge your understanding of PFCC in the context of working

Tara Lewis, Speech–Language Pathologist, Aboriginal Australian

My name is Tara Lewis. I am an Iman woman on my father's side and Yarowair on my paternal grandmother's side. As one of the youngest growing up, my ways of knowing, being, and doing within my community have largely been informed by listening and learning from the stories told by my elders and my older cousins and siblings. I grew up in Brisbane with my white mother and Aboriginal father. I remember spending a lot of my childhood with my Aboriginal cousins down by the creek and at our homes with our mob of family. Us kids we would occupy ourselves and always look after each other. We would rarely interrupt our parents or uncle's and aunty's unless it was necessary.

I didn't realize at the time, but upon reflection of my family and upbringing, we all seemed to have certain roles. The older cousins looked after the younger ones and I specifically remember my eldest male cousin putting me on his shoulders to ensure my safety as we crossed the creek. I also remember my cousins not allowing me to swing off the rope into the creek as they thought I was too little and may hurt myself. As you can imagine, I wasn't very happy! My uncle told us stories of the Junduddies to make sure we were home by dark and the responsibilities we had with looking after each other and ensuring each other's safety.

As I grew older, I was privileged with stories of my yarboo (Father) growing up. He was born in Woorabinda, an Aboriginal mission in western Queensland. Mission days sounded pretty hard and unfair particularly in the times before the 1967 Referendum when Aboriginal people were afforded political and moral rights in Australia. My yarboo spoke about the mission bell, the light-skinned children being taken away, and about the white and black schools within the missions. My Mim-Me (grandmother), yarboo, uncles, and aunties were only allowed on certain parts of the mission, and if they were caught in the prohibited areas, they were placed in jail. It didn't matter if they were kids or adults, they would still be placed in jail.

After mission days, my yarboo remembers camping by the bank of the river and foot of the mountain ranges with my great Mim-Me. He learned to track and find food in the bush, and learned about our traditional country and songlines. I remember my yarboo bringing his food tracking skills to the city, as one National Aboriginal and Islander Day Observance Committee (NAIDOC) week, he and I went down to our local park to track and find some witchetty grubs for the students at my school to taste. NAIDOC week was a big deal for us when I was at high school because it celebrates the history, culture, and achievements of Aboriginal and Torres Strait Islander people in Australia. My yarboo would help to organize activities and share his stories, and my brother would often come and teach us Aboriginal art and boomerang throwing.

My entire family has had significant involvement in informing my place and identity within my community. The value and importance of relationships and connection to place and kin have been embedded within my Iman ways of knowing, being, and doing through my elder's stories and experiences. It, however, cannot be assumed that my journey, identity, family, and community's stories equate to all Aboriginal people as a collective. My story is just one story among many.

I do, however, use my experiential knowledge as an Aboriginal speech pathologist to support my clinical practice. The first and most important component of my service is to establish a genuine and deep relationship and connection with my patients and their families. My service is rarely just about the one person that presents at the clinic for support. I ensure that I establish a genuine relationship and connection with the entire family and community they reside in. It's important for me that I have a deep and genuine understanding of the entire family and community's story and the value they hold around communication.

In order to understand the family's journey and what is important for them, I utilize "The Making Connections Framework[4]" that I helped to develop at the Institute for Urban Indigenous Health. I utilize this framework's cyclical and strengths-based approach to get connected, be connected, stay connected, and build connections with patients, families, and communities. My patient's and family's needs are at the core of my service and I ensure their needs are respected by developing an ongoing relationship based on commitment and availability for support whether it be speech–language pathology related or not.

Continued ▶

It is important to understand that speech–language pathology may not be the main concern for the patient at the time of presentation to your service. I have found on a number of occasions that some of my patients presenting to speech–language pathology often have more important challenges to attend to first. In order to determine what the priority of a patient may be, I engage in a methodology called *assessment yarning*.[5] Rather than having a list of explicit questions, somewhat like a comprehensive case history form, I yarn with my patient and his or her family through the two-way process of sharing stories. It is important that I share stories about myself and not expect my patients and their families to be the only ones sharing information. As with Aboriginal ways of communicating, it is important that the clinician shares who they are, where they are from, and who they are connected to through the methodology of *assessment yarning*.[5] This ensures a strong relational construct is formed and enables the continuation of *assessment yarning* throughout the actual assessment items.

with CALD patients and families in speech–language pathology and audiology.

Before we continue this chapter, we would first like to share some insights about being a culturally and linguistically responsive clinician from two speech–language pathologists in Australia who have different backgrounds (first, see box on previous page).

The term culture is used by different people in different contexts, to mean different things. However, for the purposes for this chapter, culture is defined as "… the shared, accumulated, and integrated set of learned beliefs, habits, attitudes, and behaviors of a group or people or community … the context in which language is developed and used and the primary vehicle by which it is transmitted".[6] In this way, CALD recognizes that groups and individuals within a population differ according to age, gender, sexual preferences, spiritual beliefs, social economic status, physical and mental capacities, geographic location, ethnicity, race, and language,[7] or because of parental identification with any of these variables.[1] Before we ask you to reflect on your own cultural values, take a moment to watch a short video featuring Sarah Verdon, an Australian speech–language pathologist; Akmaliza Ali, a Malaysian audiologist; Mansoureh Nickbakht, an Iranian audiologist; and Adrian Fuente, a Chilean audiologist, who define their own perceptions of cultural and linguistic diversity (**Video 7.1**).

Student Activity 7.1: Your Own Values and Beliefs

Just like Tara and Leanne have done, take a moment to write your own narrative about how culture has influenced your own values and beliefs as a speech–language pathology or audiology student.

A Word from a Clinical Expert: Reflections on Personal Culture

Leanne Sorbello, Speech–Language Pathologist, Italian Australian

If I reflect on my own experiences, …. I grew up in a middle-income family in Australia. My parents held strong Christian beliefs. My family is loving and supportive. I was fed, clothed, educated, and provided with strong moral guidance. My father was a Sicilian migrant and so I had exposure to family members who were raised within a different culture. I obtained a university degree, pursued a professional career as a speech–language pathologist, travelled, and acquired an illness that resulted in a below knee amputation. I married an Italian man and have two children who have been raised in a bicultural/bilingual environment. My children have thus far not had any developmental difficulties or challenging behaviors. I own a home, have a secure income, and have a happy stable home life. I have practiced as a speech–language pathologist for 26 years. All of these experiences have helped shape my personal beliefs and values. These experiences have enabled me to develop specific skills and abilities and have shaped many of my values and beliefs.

In contrast, a large number of my patients grew up within families whose cultures are not mainstream in the Australian context. Some have been raised in refugee camps and have been displaced from their cultures and extended families. Others have experienced significant traumas, chronic diseases, or have had to overcome learning difficulties. Some families have come from backgrounds of neglect and poverty, and/or have been exposed to domestic violence and various other forms of abuse. Some of the parents I work with have struggled with addiction or ongoing mental health issues. I often wonder how these experiences have shaped their own belief systems.

Just as you have reflected on how culture has influenced your own values and beliefs, two students who gained practical experience at an urban Indigenous school share their reflections on how the placement provided them with the opportunity to develop valuable knowledge of cultural considerations and sensitivities when working with patients and families who are CALD (see below).

A Word from Two Clinical Experts: Student Reflections on Their Own Culture During an Interprofessional CALD Clinic

Jacqueline Nightingale, Occupational Therapist and Madeleine Colquhoun, Speech–Language Pathologist, Australian

Throughout our time at the Australian Indigenous school, we became aware that being culturally responsive does not just mean understanding one's beliefs, traditions, and values; it is deeper than this. While it is important to consider these things, it is also important to think more broadly. As an interprofessional team, we often found we were turning our own cultural lens inward and reflecting on our own culture and history to ensure our own beliefs and values were not influencing the relationships we built with our clients and the service we were delivering. Family-centered and culturally appropriate service delivery was something our interprofessional team became passionate about while working with the children at the school and is something we will endeavor to continue implementing throughout our respective careers.

The above definition of culture also extends to groups and individuals with different sexual preferences. On next page, David Allen, an audiologist in Australia who identifies as cisgender gay man and uses he/him/his pronouns, shares some key information about how health professionals can promote positive therapeutic relationships with patients and families who identify as lesbian, gay, bisexual, or transgender (LGBT +).

In the context of working with patients who have a communication disability, it is also relevant to consider that cultural and linguistic diversity applies to patients and families from the Deaf community. Despite individuals within the Deaf community having their own cultural norms and official language, their engagement with patient- and family-centered health care services are rarely discussed.[8] In addition to ensuring that Deaf patients have access to interpreter services, there are other unique principles that need to be considered for the implementation of PFCC to Deaf patients and family members (who may also be Deaf). A recent discussion paper identified three key principles for maximizing outcomes from PFCC for Deaf patients, including (1) engaging Deaf patients in decisions about their health care; (2) developing culturally and linguistically accessible programs to support the provision of information and knowledge about health to Deaf patients; and (3) eliciting meaningful information from Deaf patients about their health care experiences, including the development of appropriate methods to measure outcomes.[8]

Before moving on to the next section, we would like you to view another video by Sarah Verdon where she describes how clinicians can be culturally responsive when working with families from a CALD background (**Video 7.2**). We also refer you to her publications on this topic[9,10] where she describes six overarching principles for working with patients who are CALD, including (1) identification of culturally appropriate and mutually motivating therapy goals; (2) knowledge of languages and culture; (3) use of culturally appropriate resources; (4) consideration of the cultural, social, and political context; (5) consultation with families and communities; and (6) collaboration between professionals.[10]

7.2 Getting Ready to be a Culturally and Linguistically Responsive Clinician

As discussed in Chapter 2, the development of optimal therapeutic relationships relies on the clinicians being cognizant of their own traditions, values, customs, and beliefs as these can influence the approach to management taken.[11] One method of increasing awareness of your own values and beliefs is through reflective practice. Reflective practice is particularly important when working with patients and families from different CALD backgrounds as this process can deepen our awareness and respect for diversity within our patient populations and help us to understand different perspectives.[11] It can also highlight existing

David Allen, Audiologist, Australian

As a health care professional, you will likely have patients and families who identify as LGBT+ . "LGBT+ " refers to a variety of people and communities, including lesbian, gay, bisexual, transgender, intersex, polyamorous, asexual, queer, pansexual, and other diverse identities. Many terms are used for these communities—you might see resources referring to "LGBTI," "LGBTIQA +," "Queer," or "Diverse in Gender and Sexuality (DiGS)" people. LGBT + people also, as a result of societal stigma, have poorer health across a range of areas, with poorer mental health outcomes, higher rates of problematic substance use, and poorer outcomes for a range of chronic health conditions.

From my perspective, I can share with you that the world can often feel like an unsafe place for LGBT + people, and this sense of insecurity can have significant impacts on how we, as clinicians, interact with our LGBT + patients and families. In particular, LGBT + people may be less likely to seek medical care for existing health issues in an attempt to avoid stigma from providers and administrative staff.

Many LGBT + people may attend health appointments in "stealth mode"—not hiding their identity per se, but simply not mentioning it or steering the conversation away from topics in which they may be forced to come out. They may choose a gender-neutral name for a partner, like "Sam" or "Ray," and refer to them as "they" to avoid being forced to choose the partner's gender. In particular, they may avoid bringing them to their own appointments. Same-sex parents may structure a child's care, so that only a single parent is ever present in an attempt to reduce the likelihood of stigma reflecting back onto their child.

This fear of stigma may also be seen in polyamorous relationships, in which more than two people enter into a committed loving relationship. Polyamorous structures can be a strong source of support and caring for their members, but may be thought of by those outside the community as "cheating," leading to a high degree of secrecy around disclosure of the structure outside the immediate family. Importantly, many polyamorous relationships involve heterosexual people, and so assumptions should not be made about a person's sexuality from the structure of his or her relationship or vice versa.

Creating an environment in which a person in a same-sex or polyamorous relationship can feel that his or her relationship is validated, can help to foster a strong therapeutic relationship, and make the partner welcome to attend and participate in the management of their communication disability. Rewriting forms to refer to "partners" or a "spouse," and reworking communication history questions to ask about "the people who you live with," "significant others," and "parents" can signal to the patient that you value and want to know about the reality of their relationships and family.

The number of people in Australia who are coming out as transgender or nonbinary, is increasing. Transgender or nonbinary persons recognize that the gender assigned to them by their doctors at birth is not accurate for them. They may more strongly identify with one or more genders, with no gender at all, or may have a gender identity that fluctuates over time. Transgender and nonbinary patients often attend speech–language pathology clinics for assistance in either feminizing or masculinizing their voices (as voice pitch and quality can be a significant source of dysphoria for them). One of the major concerns when working with transgender or nonbinary patients is "misgendering," or referring to the person as having a gender that is inaccurate for them. Misgendering a patient can be highly destructive to the therapeutic relationship. This has implications for intake forms or case history forms, and thus you may need to consider rewriting forms to refer to gender as "female," "male," or "other."

When working with transgender and nonbinary patients, it is important to recognize that your initial perception of the person's gender may not be correct, and that it is most appropriate to ask the person. Intake forms that ask patients their preferred name and what pronouns are accurate for them can be very helpful, although it may be useful to recollect this information on a semiregular basis, particularly for people actively transitioning or whose gender may be in flux. Be careful not to assume that a person's health history is related to his or her gender status—the propensity for health care professionals to make this assumption is referred to as "trans broken leg syndrome" and may lead to existing health problems being missed or ignored.

Most importantly, remember that LGBT + people do not wear signs advertising their status; there is no way, by looking at someone, to determine the person's gender or relationship status. A dear friend of mine,

Continued ▶

a semiprofessional sportsperson, told me recently about being corrected by his health professional when he referred to his partner as "he," as she did not believe that he could possibly be gay. This story reminded me, and I hope reminds you, that the most inclusive practice is one that is broad enough to accept all of our patients as they are, regardless of their sex, sexuality, gender identity, gender expression, or relationship status.

Acknowledgement: Special thanks to Elliot Harper, a transgender nonbinary person who helped with inclusive wording in this contribution.

misconceptions, assumptions, or stereotypes that we may have about patients and families from a culture different to our own and can facilitate an open and curious approach to working in a patient- and family-centered way. Importantly, speech–language pathologists and audiologists need to be free of judgement and bias when welcoming all their patients and families into the clinic, and this is especially true when the patient or family is from a CALD background. Self-reflection is never easy and requires time and practice. One way of becoming more comfortable with self-reflection is to practice it with trusted colleagues and to make it a regular part of your professional development plan. Take a moment to consider whether you have walked in your patients' shoes and whether you really know what life is like for them.

Student Activity 7.2: Reflection on How You View Patients and Families from CALD Populations

Click on the link below to access a checklist developed by American Speech–Language-Hearing Association (ASHA), and take a moment to reflect on how you view patients and families from CALD populations.

Link: https://www.asha.org/uploadedFiles/Cultural-Competence-Checklist-Personal-Reflection.pdf

7.2.1 Differences in Interactional Behaviors across Different Cultures

Across different cultures and languages, there are differences in the ways that individuals interact in both formal and informal settings, and with different communication partners. One way to acknowledge cultural and linguistic differences is to imagine for a moment that you have travelled to a country whose language you cannot speak.

Although you may think that you will be able to get by through use of nonverbal communication, such as gestures (e.g., you can always give the waiter a "thumbs up" or a nod to agree, or shake your head, or gain attention through eye contact), but when you arrive and try the gestures, you find yourself being misunderstood—or even worse—offending people. This is a good reminder that the way people interact is not universal. People from different cultures may interpret body language and gestures differently. Some gestures may mean the opposite of what you think, some may be meaningless; or there may be some gestures or eye contact that may be considered offensive.

There may also be differences in the pragmatic aspects of your communication with CALD patients and their families that relate to eye contact, physical touch, and dress. For example, some cultures will have specific customs for how female health professionals should interact with male patients and vice versa. By way of example, Mansoureh Nickbakht and Akmaliza Ali share some important insights about Iranian and Malaysian cultures that should be considered when providing speech–language pathology and audiology services to families who identify with these cultures (**Video 7.3** and excerpt later). Likewise, Adrian Fuente shares his insights about Chilean culture (**Video 7.4**).

Differences in interactional behaviors will not only be observed in nonverbal ways, but may also be observed in the narrative styles of patients and families from CALD backgrounds. This is especially important when developing effective therapeutic relationships in the delivery of PFCC. For example, in Australia, Aboriginal and Torres Strait Islander people use "yarning" as their preferred narrative style. Yarning involves the two-way sharing of stories with others who have a similar lived experience.[17] Yarning is used in Aboriginal and Torres Strait Islander culture to promote respectful and honest interactions between communication partners, and where appropriate it can be applied to any clinical interactions that speech–language pathologists and audiologists have with Aboriginal

Mansoureh Nickbakht, Audiologist, Iranian

To provide patient- and family-centered services to Iranian families who live in other countries, you may need to incorporate some cultural differences into your practice. The Iranian community is enormously diverse; while the majority of them are Persian, other ethnicities live in Iran too (e.g., Turk, Lur, Kurd, Baloch). Therefore, you may find them with entirely different points of view, educational backgrounds, and experiences. However, they may have some common characteristics that are noticeable while providing health services to them. For example, you may notice some similarities in their communication with health professionals, and in participation in decision making for their health conditions.

For good communication with an Iranian client, you may find the following strategies helpful. First, active listening will help you to build trust and rapport. Not listening to the client makes them feel disrespected that leads to miscommunication. Pleasant interaction might be even more important than your technical care for them.[12] In communication, facial expressions and appearance are also important in order to show respect.[13] Second, given that taking information is important in speech–language pathology and audiology practice, you may need to ask specific questions to gather the required information. Some Iranians might be indirect, and if asked a general question, they may not give you all the information you require. When you ask questions, they may be hesitant to say much.[14] Furthermore, they may screen the information they provide to you as they might be embarrassed to talk about some personal information.[15] You also need to give them some time to think deeply about your question. Moreover, make sure they understand the question.

In delivering the diagnosis, it is also important to consider some cultural differences as after receiving the diagnosis, people might get upset. Give them some time to digest the diagnosis. You may also begin compassionate communication with your Iranian client to give hope and optimism,[12] but just be aware of the etiquette around gender rules. For example, you may only touch people of the same gender while empathizing with them. This is also the basic etiquette for shaking hands. Shaking hands with a child is considered very respectful, while adults will not typically shake hands with people of the opposite gender.

After delivering the diagnosis, use various strategies to help your patients and their families understand the diagnosis and the importance of timely follow-up, especially as they may not want to seek professionals' help for minor health conditions.[14] You must also ask for the explicit permission from patients to deliver information about their diagnosis and treatments to other family members as some Iranians, especially the elderly, believe in protecting their loved ones (e.g., their children) from bad news and information.[16]

After building effective communication and delivering the diagnosis, it is time for decision making and its cultural considerations. As communication style is somewhat polite and indirect in Iranian culture, some clients may not be comfortable in saying "No" to people who are not close, such as health professionals. They also might be reluctant to ask many questions, so remember to check that they understand the options.[14] Some Iranian people also view health professionals as the experts and may ask them to select the best intervention for them. Therefore, clinicians should try to enhance clients' confidence so that they make the decision themselves. One way to help them feel confident enough is to provide easy-to-understand information about different aspects of each intervention. This is important as if Iranian patients do not understand the options, they may ask the health professional to select one for them or ignore the rehabilitation altogether. Another way you can increase their confidence in making decisions is to engage their family members. Family members usually take an active part in decision making about which intervention to follow.[15] Try to provide information about available options to both the patient and his or her family members who are usually wife, husband, or the eldest child.

Given that Iranians prefer to achieve quick results from the therapy, if they are not satisfied by the outcomes of the intervention, family members may encourage the patient to consider another therapist.[15] Therefore, you may consider explaining the procedures and treatment to the patients and their family members to give them realistic expectations from the intervention they selected.

Overall, given that every individual and his or her context is unique, generalizing these characteristics is not recommended. Some Iranians who live in western countries also adapt themselves to the new culture. Therefore, familiarizing ourselves with our Iranian patients would be the best approach during the service provision.

and Torres Strait Islander people. Furthermore, when western countries align with "low context" cultures wherein communication of thoughts, feelings, and ideas are more direct in comparison to other "high-context" cultures, more subtle nonverbal communication is used. As a culturally and linguistically responsive clinician, it will be important for you to recognize this and manage your own style of interaction accordingly.[2]

7.3 Planning a Culturally and Linguistically Responsive Approach to Patient- and Family-Centered Speech–Language Pathology and Audiology Services

When planning the delivery of patient- and family-centered services to a patient and his or her family from a CALD background, there are a number of additional factors that need to be considered. In **Video 7.5**, Sarah Verdon describes how the implementation of PFCC can vary across cultures.

First, you might need to consult with representatives in the community and get their advice and support about how to best engage with a member of their community. Representatives could include community leaders, parent groups, refugee services, local community health centers, and CALD support services. As a patient- and family-centered clinician, however, you will need to be cognizant of individual variability within cultural groups, as culture is not a static concept where blanket statements can be applied to an entire cultural group.[18] Thus, before making any assumptions, it is important that you consult with your patients and their families in order to seek their individual preferences regarding all aspects of their management. In addition, it might be helpful to connect with other speech–language pathologists and audiologists who have experience in providing services to families from CALD backgrounds, or who are from a different cultural or linguistic background themselves. As culturally responsive clinicians, you may also be able to support one another through special interest groups or observe each other in practice; or alternatively, engage in training or workshops on cultural responsiveness. Think about how you could integrate this into your regular professional development plan.

Leanne Sorbello's Helpful Tips

Although there are no simple answers as to how to ensure that you are culturally responsive to all your patients and their families, here are some tips:

- Be aware and sensitive. That is, use your reflective practice skills.
- Follow the patient and family's lead and avoid making assumptions based on the person's physical appearance.
- Ask experienced clinicians for their guidance.
- Take the time to do some general reading on nonverbal and interactional communication in cultures that you may frequently work with (there are many great videos and short articles online).
- Don't be afraid to ask respectfully, and learn from your patient and his or her family.
- If the family is from a non-English-speaking background, find out some keywords/phrases from them and take the time to learn them. There might also be some good resources available (e.g., for communicating with Indigenous Australians, refer to: http://www.vaccho.org.au/vcwp/wp-content/uploads/2011/03/Koorified-Aboriginal-Communication-and-Well_Being.pdf).
- Refer to ASHA's Cultural Competence Checklist for conducting culturally and linguistically appropriate services to reflect on your future speech–language pathology or audiology service (https://www.asha.org/uploadedFiles/Cultural-Competence-Checklist-Service-Delivery.pdf).

7.3.1 Consider "Who" is Family When Planning Your Service

Although we acknowledged in Chapter 1 of this book that the definition of "family" is inclusive of any person who plays a significant role in the patient's life, when working with patients and families from CALD backgrounds, the concept of family may be even broader! Patients and families from CALD backgrounds frequently live with extended family members including maternal and paternal grandparents, uncles, and aunties. In some cultures, community elders are the ones who make crucial decisions about the patient's care and, therefore, it may be expected that they need to be consulted about treatment. As a patient- and family-centered clinician, it is important to be open minded about who will make key decisions for the patient.[19] In some cultures, for example, it may be the husband or eldest son or community elder who will ultimately make the decision.

Depending on the family dynamics, different family members may accompany the patient from week to week. Sometimes the patient, be it an adult or pediatric patient, may be accompanied by a person in the family who speaks the best English, despite that person knowing very little about the patient and his or her communication disability. In this case, as a patient- and family-centered clinician, you will need to consider how to best involve that person in this capacity, and how you will involve other family members, so that you can gather and share information appropriately.

7.3.2 Consider Cultural Events When Planning Appointments

Culture and religion can have a big impact on the way you manage appointments. It may be the case that you will work with CALD families who do not keep a diary or means of recording appointments or who have fluid schedules that change on a daily basis due to changing priorities (i.e., prioritizing family commitments over clinical appointments).[20] In these cases, time management may look different to what is typically observed in a western culture. Furthermore, while our weekly timetable in western countries is traditionally organized around Monday to Friday being the working week, and Saturday and Sunday being the weekend, for some CALD patients and their families, their weeks are arranged differently. For example, for some Islamic families, Friday is the day for visiting the mosque and, therefore, may not be the best day to offer appointments. In addition, in the same way as we would never think to offer appointments to families on Christmas day, as culturally and linguistically responsive PFCC clinicians, we should be flexible and mindful of days of religious significance in other cultures.

7.3.3 Consider the Use of Interpreters and Other Supports

Being mindful of the fact that patients and families from CALD backgrounds are likely to differ in their use of the English language, one of the most important considerations for working with families from CALD backgrounds in an English-

speaking country is to understand their language preferences and requirements before they access your service. This is particularly important as communication breakdowns can impact all levels of treatment from a patient's or family member's ability to describe their health care needs to understanding their condition and what is involved in management.[1]

When your patients and their families do not have functional spoken and written English skills, you will need to seek assistance from trained interpreters or bilingual colleagues who can help interpret. Despite the increasing availability of interpreters in speech–language pathology and audiology services, a study in Canada involving 344 speech–language pathologists indicated that although 85% of respondents had access to interpreter services, less than half used them with CALD patients always or frequently.[21] It is important that interpreters are trained so that their roles and responsibilities are clearly defined and they are able to clearly communicate health care messages.[1,11] This is particularly important when practicing PFCC, as interpreters will also need to be trained in this approach (e.g., skilled in patient- and family-centered interviewing techniques).[11]

In addition, despite it sometimes being more convenient to use family members as interpreters, the evidence suggests that interpreting services are best provided by an independent person.[22] In some small communities it can be impossible to find an interpreter who is independent of the family network, and in these cases, it is not uncommon for patients and families to refuse interpreter services despite having limited English themselves. This reluctance to use an interpreter may be because in some cultures, there can be a strong sense of shame associated with communication disability and thus the patient and his or her family may not want it to be known within their network that they are accessing speech–language pathology or audiology services. If a patient and his or her family are reluctant to use an interpreter, it may be appropriate to offer the option of a phone interpreter as these interpreters often live in other cities and will therefore likely not know the patient and family. Ultimately, although we have a duty of care to ensure that health information is accurately relayed to patients and families, we also need to consider patients' and families' level of comfort with the use of interpreter services.

7.3.4 Find Out How the Values and Beliefs of the Patient's and Family's Culture May Influence Your Assessment and Management

The values and beliefs of CALD patients and their families may vary to your own, and although you may never get to a point where you completely agree with or understand these differences, as a culturally and linguistically responsive patient- and family-centered clinician, you must respect these values and beliefs. There may be differences related to their acceptance of the communication disability, differences in philosophical views related to traditional and alternative medicine, and differences in values and beliefs about family roles and responsibilities.

First, as a patient- and family-centered clinician, it is important to consider the attitudes of your patients and their families toward communication disability. In some cultures, disability may be viewed as a "failure," and therefore may not be readily accepted by the patient and/or his or her family. Conversely, in some cultures, the disability may be viewed as a retribution for previous sins, or even as part of a "divine plan." This may have implications for how you talk about the diagnosis and intervention options with your patients and families, and may require a careful and sensitive approach in all forms of communication with the patients and their immediate and broader family unit. Furthermore, the concerns of immediate family members (e.g., parents) can be undermined by extended family members whose opinions are considered to hold more value, and this can be particularly challenging when these family members have different beliefs about communication disability. Immediate family members in these situations may lack the confidence to fully describe the problem in front of extended family members or may be reluctant to seek help because of the stigma associated with the communication disability within their culture. Some cultures may even attribute blame directly to the immediate family members.[22] Great sensitivity is required and the clinician must be careful to develop an effective therapeutic relationship with the family group as a whole as opposed to just the immediate family. The provision of information and education to the family will play a key role in how the family responds to the communication disability.

In the same way that there may be differences in how CALD patients and families accept communication disability, there may also be differences in how CALD patients and families make decisions about the management of their communication disability. By way of example, despite their being inconsistent evidence, complementary and alternative medicines (CAMs) are increasingly being recognized as a treatment option for adults and children with communication disabilities.[23–26] As a culturally responsive patient- and family-centered clinician, you must remain neutral and respect your patients' decisions to seek CAMs from other practitioners. Although you might find it difficult to discuss these alternative treatments with patients and families[27] and be tempted to dismiss them as nonevidence based, as discussed in Chapter 1, evidence-based practice (EBP) must also take into consideration patient preferences and their context.

Of particular relevance to the application of PFCC in managing communication disability is the notion that patients and families may have different values and beliefs regarding their roles and responsibilities in the management process. For example, patients and families from certain cultural backgrounds may see health professionals such as speech–language pathologists and audiologists as figures of authority and people to be respected. Sometimes this means that patients and families prefer to call us "teacher" or "doctor" to show their respect. In fact, patients and families may have a stronger preference for the receipt of clinician-centered care, whereby the clinician is the key driver of care, and subsequently expect his or her speech–language pathologist or audiologist to "tell him or her what to do" and be the "expert."[19] These families can therefore be confused when we ask them to come up with treatment goals as they do not expect to have so much choice when it comes to assessment and treatment options. As a patient- and family-centered clinician, you will need to consider how the patient and the family want to be involved in goal setting, what outcomes they want to achieve, and what role they would like to play during the ongoing management of the communication disability. You may find that you need to spend a lot of time explaining the roles of different health professionals, and emphasize that you see them as the experts in their own care. In this type of situation, as long as you have practiced in a patient- and family-centered way to provide choice, in the end, patient preference for a clinician-centered approach must prevail. Later in this chapter, we will explore collaborative goal setting with CALD patients and families in more depth.

7.3.5 Preparing CALD Patients and Families for Assessment and Management

Before engaging patients and families from a CALD background in any speech–language pathology or audiology service, it is essential to first discuss with patients and families what and who will be involved in their assessment and management, and how you will work together with them. Depending on their background, CALD patients and families may not be aware of the range of health care services available and how to access these health services. Furthermore, many patients and families may have never been exposed to the types of services provided in our health care systems, and do not know what speech–language pathologists and audiologists do. For example, within Australia, there is a growing population of people from Vietnam. The first cohort of Vietnamese speech–language pathologists graduated from an Australian University in 2015, and currently there are approximately 20 speech–language pathologists to support a population of approximately 90 million people. Generations of patients with communication disability and their families have survived without ever having access to speech–language pathologists and may simply be unaware of the existence of this profession.

Moreover, in patients and families where there may have been intergenerational learning difficulties, they can bring specific prejudices or a history of negative experiences associated with the "helping" professions. For example, parents may have had numerous interventions as children, and as a result of being frequently "labeled," they may have feelings of been defined rather than being helped. These parents need reassurance that your care is likely to be different and that things have changed in regards to PFCC. For example, a strength-based approach is now best practice, and more emphasis is given to enabling a patient and his or her family to participate in their chosen contexts as opposed to fixing the problem. Patients and families, therefore, benefit from clear explanations of what is going to happen during the assessment and intervention, and they need to know about the type of care they are likely to receive. They can then make more informed decisions from the outset. Patients and families often ask the following questions:

- How much time will the therapy take?
- Tell me how to fix the problem?
- How much money will I have to spend?

Although you may not have the answer to all these questions, it is important to acknowledge this and give patients and families an indication that it is likely to take some time to get a full understanding of the patient's communication disability; however, accessing your service is the first step to addressing their needs.

7.4 Conducting a Culturally and Linguistically Responsive Speech–Language Pathology or Audiology Assessment

An important element of achieving successful outcomes for patients and their families is to conduct a comprehensive biopsychosocial assessment. When families seek help from us, we temporarily share part of their life journey. If we are going to have a positive impact on their trajectory, we must develop a thorough understanding of the patient and his or her family. As discussed in Chapter 5, your comprehensive assessment will need to involve a combination of preassessment planning, a patient- and family-centered case history, patient and family observation, patient and family self-report, and formal and informal assessment. Your preassessment planning might involve collecting some preliminary information through questionnaires, talking to other professionals, and perusing clinical notes. Importantly, you need to be mindful that patients and families may not be aware that it is appropriate to ask questions of you as their speech–language pathologist or audiologist. Encouraging them to come armed with their own set of questions is one way of being a patient- and family-centered clinician.

An example of an effective preassessment planning activity is to encourage patients and families to develop their own set of questions to ask you at the first appointment as a starting point for assessment and intervention. Patients and families can come up with broad questions such as What is wrong with my hearing? How can I help my child to talk better? Is my child developing like other children of his or her age? Why doesn't my husband realize how his language problems are affecting me? Sometimes patient and family questions are based on what other people have told them or what they have read on the internet. A frequent question may be "Does my child have autism?" The purpose of starting from patient and family questions is to ensure that the voices of patients and families are clearly heard so that their needs can be fully addressed.

As patients and families from CALD backgrounds can find it challenging to generate their own questions, question prompt lists (QPLs) are increasingly being used by health professionals to give patients and families a helping hand. Although these QPLs have primarily been utilized in medicine,[28] their application to speech–language pathology and audiology is emerging. One example that can be used with all parents of children with hearing loss by speech–language pathologists and audiologists is available at http://alliedweb.s3.amazonaws.com/hearingr/diged/201711/index.html.[29] More generic QPLs can be found on the Agency for Healthcare Research and Quality website https://www.ahrq.gov/patients-consumers/patient-involvement/ask-your-doctor/index.html.

Use the Question Builder on the Agency for Healthcare Research and Quality website, https://www.ahrq.gov/patients-consumers/question-builder.html. practice generating your own list of questions for an upcoming health appointment for either yourself or a family member.

In Chapter 5, we discussed, very broadly, the types of questions that should be incorporated into a patient- and family-centered case history to ensure you gather information about the patient's and family's biopsychosocial functioning. When working with patients and families from a CALD background, there may be some additional considerations for how you ask these questions and additional questions that may be required. A good rule of thumb is to observe patients and families closely. As a culturally and linguistically responsive clinician, you should approach your case history interview gently, perhaps starting with a set of generic open-ended questions about their life or why they have come to see you. Some examples of these questions are given below:

- *Is there anything that is particularly troubling you?*
- *Tell me what a typical day is like for you or your family?*
- *What would you like to know about your child's development?*
- *How can I be of assistance to you?*

The use of open questions also encourages more open conversation that resembles "story telling" and also allows patients and families to share as much or as little information that they feel comfortable sharing. How patients and families react to these open questions will provide us with cues to proceed with our case history questions. It is important to remember that some questions and information can be left until you have developed an effective therapeutic relationship with your patients and their families. Getting advice and training on how to ask difficult questions or broach sensitive topics is an important aspect of our role. A number of other professionals, for example, psychologists and social workers have specific training in discussing sensitive issues with patients and families, and they can be a valuable source of support in any workplace. Generally speaking, the use of direct questioning is only appropriate when seeking basic information from patients and families but should otherwise be avoided.

As Tara Lewis reflected earlier, before seeking personal information from patients and families, a good strategy is to disclose something personal about yourself first. This can ease the pressure on patients and families, and potentially make them feel more comfortable to share their story. Another consideration is to not be afraid of "silences" in your case history interview. Pausing throughout your assessment can also make patients and their families feel more comfortable. Do not rush to fill the silence.

I once worked with a child who had lived in four countries and been exposed to eight languages before the age of 8 years. Her parents had experienced many traumas before arriving in Australia including threat of death, periods where it was difficult to find food, and instances of physical and sexual abuse. They were in Australia on a temporary protection visa. The 8 year old had learning and language difficulties, and she suffered ongoing chronic headaches and allergies. Medically, the child was diagnosed with a rare syndrome that should have been detected at a much younger age. The family spoke very little English, lived in public housing (three bedrooms for seven family members), and were experiencing mental health issues.

~ Leanne Sorbello, Speech–Language Pathologist, Italian-Australian

This story shared by Leanne is just one of many stories you are likely to hear when working with patients and families who are CALD. Therefore, the case history interview you conduct with patients and families from CALD backgrounds may be complex. It is important that you approach it with insight and sensitivity and gather additional information about their beliefs, concerns, and reasons for seeking help, especially as these may differ from the general population.[11] ▶ Fig. 7.1 provides an outline of suggested case history questions you could include when working with CALD patients and their families.

Case history question	Rationale
CALD background	Detailed information should be gathered about the patient and family's CALD background, including: • country of birth • length of time living in current country • other countries lived in • cultures that the family identifies with
Patient and family educational background	It is important to understand the literacy and language levels of patients and families as this will shape how we will present information and resources. It may be necessary to keep messages short and simple for these families to help them engage with your service.
Family dynamics	CALD families may have a larger extended family: and diversity' in family dynamics such that more senior family may "carry more weight" and can be very influential in how patients and families perceive the communication disability'. Extended family may also play a more central role in goal setting and intervention planning.
Language profile	CALD patients and families may have been exposed to multiple languages and cultures, therefore it is essential to have some understanding of the following: • pattern of language exposure for the child • the level of English spoken and understood by caregivers • the patient and family's language preferences for their home language and English • the patient and family's beliefs about language learning and its relationship to educational outcomes (i.e.,: do they think that if their child does not speak English before they go to school, that this child will be disadvantaged?)
Trauma experiences	Speech-language pathologists and audiologists may work with patients and families who are migrants or asylum seekers. These patients and families may have been itinerant for many years or spent much of their lives in detention or refugee camps.
Family values and beliefs	Some information about the family of origin of parents coming to our service can be useful. This provides information on how supported the parents may be in caring for their children but also whether they themselves have had positive role models. This enables a deeper understanding of belief and value systems around parenting practises. Understand what parents believe about their role can help us to empower them to make changes.
Consideration of communicative competence in native language	Ask patients and their families about the patient's exposure to English and their native languages and their language developmental history.

Fig. 7.1 Suggested case history questions for working with CALD populations in speech–language pathology and audiology.

In Chapter 5, you completed a student activity whereby you extended a "standard" case history to include biopsychosocial questions. Now, we would like you to extend this even further! Work in pairs and develop five questions you could ask patients and their family members from a CALD background which will build your knowledge and understanding of their cultural and linguistic background.

Once you have the list of CALD case history questions, take turns in playing the role of the clinician and the patient and/or family member. When acting as the clinician, challenge yourself to do more listening than talking!

Reflect on how you felt as both clinician and patient/family member. Were you comfortable? What was hard and what was easy?

In terms of assessment batteries, when conducting formal assessments, you will need to consider the availability of assessments which are culturally and linguistically appropriate. For example, you need to consider whether there are translations available, if the assessments have culturally appropriate normative data, and whether the assessments diagnose a deficit or a difference in your patient's communication skills. As there is often a lack of culturally and linguistically appropriate assessment tools in speech–language pathology and audiology,[30] more often than not, you will find the use of patient and family observation, informal language samples, dynamic assessment, and patient, family, and other self- and proxy-report as key to informing your overall diagnosis. Throughout all aspects of your assessment, you will need to consider in what language you will assess the patient's communicative functioning, and indeed may need to assess in both their home language and English.[11] In the right column box, Jacqueline and Madeleine describe their experiences of conducting a culturally and linguistically responsive assessment while on a student placement at an urban Indigenous school.

Jacqueline Nightingale, Occupational Therapist and Madeleine Colquhoun, Speech–Language Pathologist, Australian
While delivering interprofessional clinics at the school, we were fortunate enough to have the opportunity to participate in dynamic assessment and intervention as a part of an interprofessional team. As a team, we quickly became aware of the importance of choosing assessment methods and interventions that were appropriate to the cultural group we were working with. We gained an understanding that standardized assessment does not always take into consideration one's cultural values with the standardized score not truly encompassing one's abilities. Therefore, in order to deliver culturally responsive practice, we became aware of the importance of choosing assessment methods that reflect the cultural and social background of the children we were working with. As such, it was our responsibility to plan assessment and intervention sessions as an interprofessional team that were flexible, patient- and family-centered, engaging, and culturally appropriate, and which provided us with the information we required.

7.4.1 Developing a Shared Understanding of the Problem

An important aspect of working with patients and families from CALD backgrounds is to consider how the patients and families themselves perceive the communication disability. At this time, it is useful to establish the level of patient and family concern, and how the patients and their families describe the problem. Sometimes, the patients and families themselves have not initially identified a problem with communication functioning, rather, it was identified by someone else in their environment (e.g., a child health nurse, a general practitioner, a teacher, an employer, or a friend).

There may be a number of reasons why patients and families have not recognized the presence of a communication disability. For example, people from diverse cultural or linguistic backgrounds may have different expectations of communicative functioning informed by their cultural beliefs and experiences. Health professionals often talk about overutilizing public resources to service the "worried well." When working with patients and families from CALD backgrounds, the opposite can be true, whereby a larger proportion of patients and families could be defined as the "unworried unwell." It is sometimes the case that with intergenerational developmental difficulties and pervasively poor learning outcomes across a community, general expectations of communicative functioning can be lower. As one's communicative development is often compared to others in the same community who may also be experiencing communication disability, these observations can be misleading and suggest to the patient and/or family that the patient is functioning well, when they are actually experiencing a communication delay or disorder. Another reason why patients and families may not recognize a communication disability is due to bilingualism.

When patients and families do not identify a communication problem, an ethical conundrum is thrown up for the speech–language pathologist or audiologist. If a patient and his or her family are happy and take pride in what existing skills the patient has, then the role of the clinician in providing a more realistic picture of their communicative functioning can be a negative experience for the patient and his or her family, and a threat for the development of an effective patient–family–clinician therapeutic relationship. In this case, a key role of the speech–language pathologist or audiologist will be to sensitively provide some general information and education around communication development and functioning. In the case of pediatric patients, if you find that parents are not readily acknowledging their child's communication disability, it can be helpful to address potential feelings of parental guilt and reassure parents that it is not always possible to attribute a single cause to communication disability, and importantly, they are not to blame.

7.4.2 Sharing Assessment Results in a Culturally and Linguistically Responsive Manner

Once we have completed our assessments, it is important to dedicate some time to explaining the results of the assessment with the family. Sometimes this involves giving a diagnosis and/or referring the patient and family onto another health professional. Providing feedback on assessment results to patients and families from CALD backgrounds can be particularly challenging because the problem and the cause can be multilayered and complex. Sometimes it can be better to provide small amounts of information at a time and build the bigger picture over a longer period of time. Let the patients and families be your guide and regularly check in with them to see how they feel. Be prepared to revisit questions or address new questions as they arise. If interpreters are involved, it is often best to meet with the interpreter before sharing assessment results to ensure that the message you are going to send is both sensitive and accurate. If you are making a diagnosis, explore ways of defining the name of the diagnosis in the second language that is meaningful to the family but not too insensitive.

It is never easy to predict how patients and families will react when you share assessment information and provide feedback on the communication disability. A lot depends on the patient's and family's initial understanding of the communication disability. Some patients and families may indicate that they are relieved when they finally have a label for the communication disability. Other patients

"I was once very anxious about giving some bad news to a family. They surprised me by responding in a very philosophical manner. They shrugged their shoulders and said "well we have done nothing wrong. If this is what the Lord has given us then we must accept it and do the best we can to help this child. What can we do to help her?"

~ Leanne Sorbello, Speech–Language Pathologist, Italian-Australian

and families on the other hand are fearful of labels as they may carry a stigma and wish for that information to remain confidential and may not want to share the assessment results with others, including other health professionals, teachers, employers, etc.

When you provide a diagnosis, patients and families may experience feelings of grief and loss, so it is always good to have a box of tissues surreptitiously but strategically placed when sharing assessment results. Patients and families may cry. As you may feel uncomfortable when this happens, you could try simply sitting with patients and families in their sadness. More often than not, the patient and family will be the first to lift the mood and move on. Sometimes families and parents cry because they have not been heard and not because they have been hurt by your comments. Some patients and families from CALD backgrounds have held things together for so long, within a lot of adversity, that the moment someone acknowledges their challenges, it triggers an emotional release. Other times, patients and families may respond with anger and frustration or simply disagree with the assessment results. These patients and families respond best by being listened to. Listening quietly and acknowledging can defuse situations. When patients and families are angry, they may not have the capacity to hear and will need time to work through their emotions. It is important to salvage the therapeutic relationship over being right. For some patients and families, anger is their only way of dealing with adverse situations, and it is rarely anything personal.

As a patient- and family-centered clinician, it is important that you explicitly acknowledge and build on the strengths of both the patient and the family. In doing this, you may very well be the first health professional that the patient and family have come into contact with who has provided some positive feedback about the patient's functioning. When you highlight their strengths, you might find that vulnerable patients and families will quickly warm to you and become filled with a sense of pride. The happiness they feel when you praise some aspects of their communicative and family functioning is palpable. This does not mean that you are diminishing the patient's difficulties, rather you are building a platform on which to resolve the difficulties. Focusing on deficits alone is not conducive to being a patient- and family-centered clinician, nor does it empower patients and families to create change. We have to be realistic about prognosis, but we should not deny patients and families the opportunity of seeing the potential for change and improvement. Taking this strengths-based perspective is a powerful way of developing an effective patient–family–clinician therapeutic relationship, and this will ultimately lead to better outcomes for the patient and his or family. Some basic principles for sharing assessment results in a culturally and linguistically responsive manner are outlined in ▸ Fig. 7.2.

7.5 Culturally and Linguistically Responsive Approaches to Collaborative Management Planning

7.5.1 Collaborative Goal Setting and Decision Making with CALD Patients and Families

Once we have identified and understood the patient's communication disability, we naturally need to address the biopsychosocial needs of patients and their families. The initial phase of intervention usually involves developing collaborative goals with the patients and their families that best align with their own beliefs and priorities.[2] The concept of setting a goal is interesting, and some health professionals describe goal setting as a "first world concept." You may find that some patients and families from CALD backgrounds have never set a goal in their life and in fact may not necessarily think about the future. Furthermore, patients and families who are from cultures where it is expected that the health professional be the one to decide on goals can be very anxious or confused about what to do. As a result, the process of collaborative goal setting may be challenging for some CALD patients and families. Therefore, it is even more paramount that you explicitly explain the joint process behind goal setting, and importantly give families time to think about goals before they come in for the session.

Principle	Strategies
Feedback should be tailored to meet the needs of the family	Providing too much information about the patient's communication difficulties can be overwhelming for CALD patients and families. The feedback you provide and the way you deliver it should be individualized. Consider: • How might the feedback impact on the patient and family emotionally? • Is my message going to be well accepted by the patient and family? • How easy will it be for the patient and family to understand what I have to say? Structure feedback around a few key messages, prioritizing the type of information you share. Consider: • What is having the most impact on the patient and family? • What is most important to the patient and family (this could be linked to their questions)?
Feedback should be adapted to meet the capacity of the family	As patients and families who are CALD may experience difficulty understanding language, it is helpful to use supportive communication strategies to deliver feedback. This could involve: • Providing written information in easy English. • Simplifying explanations as much as possible. • Providing concrete examples from the assessment. • Using graphics and pictures - but do not turn feedback into a tutorial. • Using the patient and family's own words to describe things. • Wait for the patient or family to make a comment or ask questions. Give families more thinking time by allowing pauses. • Make sure families understand that no question is a silly question.
Feedback should be non-judgemental	When sharing assessment results with patients and families from CALD backgrounds, it is important that we: • Do our best to see things from the patient and family's perspective. • Be disciplined to make sure that our personal opinions are not in any way reflected in our words.

Fig. 7.2 Principles for sharing assessment results in a culturally and linguistically responsive manner.

A Helpful Tip

It is useful for speech–language pathologists and audiologists to develop skills in training patients and families to set goals and implement action plans. It can be helpful to ask families to think about aspects of their life (e.g., home, community, work, school), and think where help is needed the most. Ask them to think about the hows and whys of communication, what the patient can do, and what the next step should be. Ask questions such as "What are the things that you do sometimes and how can we make this happen more often?"

Commercial tools are available that can help patients and families set goals. For example, patients and families can sort through cards depicting different life situations in picture and word form and sort them into "now," "maybe later," and "not a priority at all" categories. These tools will help patients and families prioritize.

Once you have established some clear goals with CALD patients and families, it is important to engage them in the decision making process about longer-term management options. Research suggests that families from CALD backgrounds may have difficulty in engaging in shared decision making, identifying their role in management, and taking action.[2] In addition to the obvious language barriers, patients and families from CALD backgrounds can have less trust in health care systems and providers, and thus may be less willing to share preferences and values while engaging in the shared decision making process.[19] This means that in order to practice PFCC with patients and families from CALD backgrounds, you will need to draw on your entire suite of patient- and family-centered skills, including the creation of a safe environment where your patients and families feel validated and an integral part of the team. You will need to use effective communication strategies to ensure patients and families have a clear understanding of the entire situation by explaining what

A Word from a Clinical Expert: Reflections on Establishing Patient- and Family-Centered Management Plans with Singaporeans

Brena Lim, Speech–Language Pathologist, Singaporean

Singapore is a multinational and multicultural country comprising many different races and people from different nationalities. As Singaporean society has evolved, health care has moved from a medical or impairment-based model to a collaborative and therapeutic model that is centered around the patient, family, and clinician. This has resulted in the development of multiple forms of service delivery that are used to deliver PFCC.

As a speech–language pathologist, it all starts with obtaining a case history from the patient. For multilingual clinicians, building rapport and developing a trusting and respectful therapeutic relationship might be as simple as speaking in the patient's and family's preferred language. With the building of rapport comes knowledge of the family dynamics. As a speech–language pathologist, one of the main things I have learnt is to respect each family's unique structure. For example, if I am working with a traditional Chinese/Asian family who may have a greater preference for clinician-centered care, I will ask the family to participate and help with rehabilitation for the patient. I will specifically ask the family to develop a list of words that are associated with the patient's or family's likes, dislikes, or hobbies. I might also focus on words that the family want the patient to relearn for a social gathering (e.g., Chinese New Year). In contrast, for a family that is more independent, and predominantly westernized in its thinking, I will encourage the patient and family to set goals for themselves.

The approach to management will usually be determined based on a family conference that involves the patient, family, doctors, and clinicians. Although the doctors and clinicians typically chair this conference, management directions, the potential for rehabilitation, and the development of suitable goals will be discussed with the patient and the family. Within clinical sessions, I initially involve families by asking them to observe the session. This not only assists in developing trust and rapport, but also develops family confidence in conducting therapy tasks themselves. The session should be conducted in the language that is preferred by both the patient and the family.

you do and are doing, using clear and easy-to-understand language, checking their understanding by asking questions, and encouraging them to ask questions. It can be helpful to write down instructions that can be taken home, avoid the use of jargon, and use the patient's and family's own words where possible.[2]

As described in Chapter 6, decision aids are a commonly used method for promoting shared decision making in health care. However, caution must be taken when using decision aids with CALD patients and families when an interpreter service is required. In particular, clinicians have been shown to have difficulty conveying the full picture regarding intervention options when working with interpreters, and interpreters who are not trained in the principles of PFCC and shared decision making may find it difficult to convey these options in a truly unbiased manner.[31] Therefore, when using tools to promote shared decision making with CALD patients and families, it is necessary that you explain the rationale and process of using a decision aid to your patients and families.

In the above box, Brena Lim, a Singaporean speech–language pathologist, shares her experiences with setting goals and planning interventions with different cultural groups within Singapore.

7.5.2 Considerations for the Delivery of Culturally and Linguistically Responsive Services

When considering models of service delivery for patients and families from CALD backgrounds, there are a number of factors which you need to consider. One of the key considerations in the delivery of culturally and linguistically responsive health care services is to create a welcoming environment where information is readily available in both English and languages of the local community.[11] Specifically, as discussed in Chapter 3, written health information should be provided for patients and families at a reading grade level lower than 6. This is particularly important when working with CALD patients and families who do not have English as a first language, and thus may have even lower levels of written health literacy compared to the general population. Translations of written health information into the patient's and family's home language may also be required.[11] Furthermore, any resources which you use should contain culturally appropriate language, pictures, concepts, and content in order to ensure the clinical environment is safe and welcoming for patients and families.[11] It is also important to be aware of the increasing number of resources which have been made available in different languages, and even if your patients and their families have good English, they often appreciate being offered the option of having resources provided in their first language.

Think about an area of clinical practice that you most enjoy working in. Research what translated resources are available for that area of practice, and share that resource with another student.

In regard to service delivery models, while it may seem simpler to provide individual in-clinic services to CALD patients and their families, especially if they do not have functional English, this should not rule out the possibility of other models of service delivery, which provide more naturalistic contexts, such as groups, mobile services, and telepractice.[11] In ▶ Fig. 7.3, Cindy Smith, a Canadian speech–language pathologist, has provided some top tips for working with families and young children from CALD backgrounds in groups.

Before offering mobile services such as home visits to CALD populations, it is essential to check if this model of service delivery is culturally appropriate for the patient and family, and whether there is anything that you should know about before you visit. For example, if you are a female entering an Islamic household, you will need to be very aware of the dress code, as it would not be culturally responsive to make patients and their

Tip	How could they apply to your practice?
1 Find out how the assessment and intervention approach fits with the philosophy of the patient and family's culture.	If a pediatric patient comes from a culture where children traditionally do what they are told to do by adults, may find child-centered language stimulation strategies such as 'Let the child lead' and 'Follow the child's lead' challenging. It doesn't mean you can't still do it, but you'll need to be very clear on why, and what the limitations are. I often talk about 'Letting the child lead' as being 'Let the child show you what they are interested in'.
2 Consult with representatives in the community and get their advice and support.	Representatives could include community leaders, parent groups, refugee services, local community health, and CALD support services in the community.
3 Check if the family's English is sufficient to understand what is being said.	Check this beforehand as you may lose the family part way through the program otherwise. It may be best to work with families who do not have functional English 1:1, allowing greater flexibility for the level of input and speed of presentation. If you feel a family really wants to attend the group sessions but may be challenged by the language level, ensure they have adequate pre-reading/watching materials and be prepared to revisit the strategies in more detail during the individual sessions.
4 Find out what translations are available.	Even if people have good English they often really appreciate resources in their first language.
5 Consider how the use of interpreters will impact your group dynamics.	It's hard to use more than one interpreter per group; the interpreter should be trained in what you are delivering; and you will need to allow more time.
6 Ensure parents are clear on the basics of the group functioning.	Examples are: adults only at the groups, must be the same adult each week, and must adhere to group etiquette.
7 Consider the attitudes of extended family.	Extended family members who have a different attitude and approach may wield a fair amount of influence, even with parents who are very 'on board' about the approach. Think about holding an information session for extended family and/or providing additional resources.
8 Think about adapting the strategies somewhat for cultures who may be challenged by some of the material.	For example, if play isn't part of a family's culture, you could talk about how to incorporate play into daily routines, such as: nappy changing and bath time such that they do not need to instigate a separate play activity.
9 Try and connect with other speech pathologists who have provided services for families from CALD backgrounds.	Support one another in special interest groups or observe each other in practice. This will encourage information sharing.

Fig. 7.3 Cindy Smith's Top Tips for working with CALD populations in speech–language pathology and audiology.

Teresa Quinlan, Occupational Therapist, American and Anne Hill, Speech–Language Pathologist, Australian

The University of Queensland occupational therapy and speech–language pathology clinical educators and students participate in a weekly interprofessional clinic at an urban Indigenous school for students from prep to year 12. This clinic has been built from strong foundations. First, a successful model for interprofessional clinics has been implemented within The University of Queensland Health and Rehabilitation Clinics for many years.[32] This model focusses on exposure to, development of, and reflection on interprofessional processes and collective ownership of client goals. Second, the interprofessional clinic evolved in 2011 from a long-standing occupational therapy clinic conducted at the school since 1997. Students work in interprofessional teams at the school for a half day/week for 12 weeks during each university semester to work with school staff to support children's skills for school participation and learning. Programs are strengths based and incorporate activities with cultural meaning and functional significance for children and families.[33]

Research with students and clinical educators in this clinic has identified factors and approaches that support student learning of cultural responsiveness and interprofessional practice skills and facilitate positive outcomes for clients.[33,34] The themes identified in this research echo the components identified in the PFCC model proposed in this book: effective clinician–patient–family relationships, the incorporation of patient and family needs, and patient- and family-driven care.

Within our clinic, we highlight and enact a range of models that can help students to understand themselves, each other, the context and, most importantly, the clients. In particular, we draw on Indigenous Allied Health Australia's (IAHA) Cultural Responsiveness in Action Framework,[35] the International Classification of Functioning, Disability and Health (ICF),[36] the Canadian National Interprofessional Competency Framework,[37] the Kawa model,[38] and the Person-Environment-Occupation Model (PEO).[39] These are introduced and reiterated in the clinic and provide a foundation for students' client-centered planning and clinical reasoning and their own self-evaluation.

Our commitment to nourishing relationships within the school community is evidenced in how we structure the clinic. Frequent planning meetings are scheduled prior to the start of the clinic to discuss the needs of the children and how we can best support them. Intentional and focused time to build relationships and listen to the needs of the school allow us the opportunity to prioritize the assessments and interventions that meet the changing needs of the school community. A strengths-based approach is integrated into all aspects of our interprofessional clinical teaching, and we have found the PEO model valuable in supporting our students' understanding of the whole person during this process. This is a dynamic model that encourages our students to consider the changing relationship between the children, their roles within the context of school, home, and community (a learner, friend, and sibling), and the impact the environment (school, home, and social situations) has on their self-identity and engagement in life skills.

By encouraging students to always focus on how their planned therapy sessions will impact the children, they are supported to develop more culturally appropriate ways of assessment and intervention, including the use of "yarning" to engage children, build a positive relationship, and gain more valid information.[5] The Kawa model[38] is a culturally relevant model that allows clients a platform to tell their story. It uses the metaphor of a river and describes the client's daily life (including strengths and struggles) as life flow. We have found this model helpful in providing our students with a structure to build relationships and "have a yarn" with their clients. Taking time to listen to the child's story and work in collaboration with the child, teacher, and school community fosters a relationship that is client-centered and culturally responsive.

Clinic processes have been trialled and revised over the years to support this collaborative practice within the school environment. For example, we have structured an orientation program that includes members of the school community sharing cultural perspectives and stories with our student teams. Icebreaker and teambuilding activities provide our students opportunities to share personal and professional experiences. Our student teams work side by side from the first week in planning, resourcing, documentating, and debriefing. Journal club and morning teas are scheduled weekly to provide an opportunity to build relationships and facilitate professional discussion around clinical, cultural, and interprofessional development.

Our leadership in interprofessional reasoning and team building and in collaborative practice with the clients, the staff, and the school community support students in recognizing that interprofessional practice allows us to provide an effective patient-centered and culturally responsive service.

families feel uncomfortable. Another consideration for mobile services is etiquette around the acceptance of food and drink. While you may think it is more appropriate to decline food and drink on home visits, in some cultures where it is customary for the family to offer food or drink, it may be considered rude to decline the offer. It is important to be aware of cultural norms before deciding whether to accept or not. For example, in some homes, you may find yourself being brought a cup of juice without being asked, as a culturally appropriate way of welcoming visitors.

As a student speech–language pathologist or audiologist, it is likely you will have an opportunity to experience a CALD clinical placement. See the box on previous page, Teresa Quinlan and Anne Hill describe how they prepare students so that they can benefit the most from this type of placement. You might also find these tips helpful when preparing for a CALD placement.

7.6 Bringing It All Together

In this chapter, we have introduced you to the different aspects of speech–language pathology and audiology practice that can be influenced by cultural and linguistic diversity. We have discussed a number of key supports and resources which can overcome barriers to providing culturally and linguistically responsive patient- and family-centered services, including (1) the use of interpreters; (2) the availability of CALD clinicians; (3) the use of assessments in the patient's and family's home language; (4) the consideration of "normative" data in the patient's home language; (5) your own cultural knowledge; and (6) the importance of reflective practice and professional development for working with CALD patients and families.[21] Although we have only scratched the surface of this complex and clinically important work, as a patient- and family-centered clinician in training, we hope this has inspired you to expand your learning as you get ready to be a culturally and linguistically responsive clinician capable of modifying your assessment and management to meet the needs of your patients and families from CALD backgrounds. To end with, take a moment to watch one last video by Sarah Verdon where she provides advice for working with families from a CALD background you are not familiar with (**Video 7.6**).

7.7 Reflections

Please respond to the following reflection questions in your PFCC journal:
1. How might "family" be different for patients from CALD backgrounds?
2. What is a QPL and how might it be used in the assessment of patients and families from CALD backgrounds?
3. Consider a recent speech–language pathology or audiology clinical session you participated in where the patient and his or her family came from a different culture than your own. How did this session compare with other clinical encounters where you and the patient share the same culture? Were there any challenges and if so how did you manage these?

References

[1] Komaric N, Bedford S, van Driel ML. Two sides of the coin: patient and provider perceptions of health care delivery to patients from culturally and linguistically diverse backgrounds. BMC Health Serv Res. 2012; 12(1):322

[2] King G, Desmarais C, Lindsay S, Piérart G, Tétreault S. The roles of effective communication and client engagement in delivering culturally sensitive care to immigrant parents of children with disabilities. Disabil Rehabil. 2015; 37(15):1372–1381

[3] Hasnain R, Kondratowicz DM, Borokhovski E, et al. Do Cultural Competency Interventions Work? A Systematic Review on Improving Rehabilitation Outcomes for Ethnically and Linguistically Diverse Individuals with Disabilities. Vol 31. Austin, TX: National Center for the Dissemination of Disability Research; 2011

[4] Nelson A, McLaren C, Lewis T, Iwama M. Cultural influences and occupation-centred practice with children and families. In: Rodgers S, ed. Occupation-Centred Practice with Children: A Practical Guide for Occupational Therapists. 2nd ed. West Sussex: Wiley and Sons; 2017:73–89

[5] Lewis T, Hill A, Bond C, Nelson A. Yarning: assessing proppa ways. J Clin Pract Speech Lang Pathol. 2017; 19(1):14–18

[6] Kohnert K. Language Disorders in Bilingual Children and Adults. San Diego, CA: Plural Publishers; 2008. https://www.mhahs.org.au/images/cald/CulturalCompetencyInHealth.pdf. Accessed March 15, 2019

[7] Australian Government National Health and Medical Research Council. Cultural Competency in Health: A Guide for Policy, Partnerships, and Participation. Commonwealth of Australia. 2006

[8] Rogers KD, Ferguson-Coleman E, Young A. Challenges of realising patient-centred outcomes for Deaf patients. Patient. 2018; 11(1):9–16

[9] Verdon S, Wong S, McLeod S. Shared knowledge and mutual respect: enhancing culturally competent practice through collaboration with families and communities. Child Lang Teach Ther. 2016; 32(2):205–221

[10] Verdon S, McLeod S, Wong S. Supporting culturally and linguistically diverse children with speech, language and

communication needs: overarching principles, individual approaches. J Commun Disord. 2015; 58:74–90

[11] Australia SP. Working in a Culturally and Linguistically Diverse Society: Clinical Guideline; 2016. https://www.speech-pathologyaustralia.org.au/SPAweb/Members/Clinical_Guidelines/spaweb/Members/Clinical_Guidelines/Clinical_Guidelines.aspx?hkey=f66634e4-825a-4f1a-910d-644553f59140. Accessed March 15, 2019

[12] Martin SS. Healthcare-seeking behaviors of older Iranian immigrants: health perceptions and definitions. J Evid Based Soc Work. 2009; 6(1):58–78

[13] Ebrahimi H, Torabizadeh C, Mohammadi E, Valizadeh S. Patients' perception of dignity in Iranian healthcare settings: a qualitative content analysis. J Med Ethics. 2012; 38(12):723–728

[14] Behati-Sabet A, Chambers NA. People of Iranian descent. In: Waxler-Morrison N, Anderson JM, Richardson E, Chambers NA, eds. Cross-Cultural Caring: A Handbook for Health Professionals. 2nd ed. Vancouver: UBC Press; 2011:127–161

[15] Jalali B. Iranian family. In: McGoldrick M, Giordano J, Garcia-Preto N, eds. Ethnicity and Family Therapy. 3rd ed. New York, NY: Guilford Publications; 2005:451–467

[16] HealthCare Chaplaincy. A Dictionary of Patients' Spiritual & Cultural Values for Health Care Professionals. 2010; http://www.healthcarechaplaincy.org/userimages/Cultural%20&%20Spiritual%20Dictionary%2012-20-10.pdf. Accessed November 28, 2018

[17] Geia LK, Hayes B, Usher K. Yarning/aboriginal storytelling: towards an understanding of an Indigenous perspective and its implications for research practice. Contemp Nurse. 2013; 46(1):13–17

[18] Almutairi AF, Dahinten VS, Rodney P. Almutairi's Critical Cultural Competence model for a multicultural healthcare environment. Nurs Inq. 2015; 22(4):317–325

[19] Hawley ST, Morris AM. Cultural challenges to engaging patients in shared decision making. Patient Educ Couns. 2017; 100(1):18–24

[20] Sotnik P, Jezewski MA. Culture and disability services. In: Stone JH, ed. Culture and Disability: Providing Culturally Competent Services. Thousand Oaks, CA: SAGE; 2005:15–36

[21] D'Souza C, Bird E, Deacon H. Survey of Canadian speech-language pathology service delivery to linguistically diverse clients. Can J Speech Lang Pathol Audiol. 2012; 36(1):18–39

[22] Stow C, Dodd B. Providing an equitable service to bilingual children in the UK: a review. Int J Lang Commun Disord. 2003; 38(4):351–377

[23] Laures J, Shisler R. Complementary and alternative medical approaches to treating adult neurogenic communication disorders: a review. Disabil Rehabil. 2004; 26(6):315–325

[24] Lewanda AF, Gallegos MF, Summar M. Patterns of dietary supplement use in children with Down syndrome. J Pediatr. 2018; 201:100–105.e30

[25] Şenel HG. Parents' views and experiences about complementary and alternative medicine treatments for their children with autistic spectrum disorder. J Autism Dev Disord. 2010; 40(4):494–503

[26] Yiu E, Xu JJ, Murry T, et al. A randomized treatment-placebo study of the effectiveness of acupuncture for benign vocal pathologies. J Voice. 2006; 20(1):144–156

[27] Hall H, Brosnan C, Frawley J, Wardle J, Collins M, Leach M. Nurses' communication regarding patients' use of complementary and alternative medicine. Collegian. 2018; 25(3):285–291

[28] Brown RF, Bylund CL, Li Y, Edgerson S, Butow P. Testing the utility of a cancer clinical trial specific Question Prompt List (QPL-CT) during oncology consultations. Patient Educ Couns. 2012; 88(2):311–317

[29] English K, Walker E, Farah K, et al. Implementing family-centered care in early intervention for children with hearing loss: engaging parents with a Question Prompt List (QPL). Hearing Review. 2017; 24(11):12–18

[30] McLeod S, Verdon S, Bowen C, International Expert Panel on Multilingual Children's Speech. International aspirations for speech–language pathologists' practice with multilingual children with speech sound disorders: development of a position paper. J Commun Disord. 2013; 46(4):375–387

[31] Wood F, Phillips K, Edwards A, Elwyn G. Working with interpreters: The challenges of introducing Option Grid patient decision aids. Patient Educ Couns. 2017; 100(3):456–464

[32] Copley JA, Allison HD, Hill AE, Moran MC, Tait JA, Day T. Making interprofessional education real: a university clinic model. Aust Health Rev. 2007; 31(3):351–357

[33] Hill AE, Nelson A, Copley J, Quinlan T, White R. Development of student clinics in Indigenous contexts: what works? J Clin Pract Speech Lang Pathol. 2017; 19(1):40–45

[34] Davidson B, Hill AE, Nelson A. Responding to the World Report on Disability in Australia: lessons from collaboration in an urban Aboriginal and Torres Strait Islander school. Int J Speech-Language Pathol. 2013; 15(1):69–74

[35] Indigenous Allied Health Australia. Cultural Responsiveness in Action Framework. Deakin, ACT: IAHA; 2015

[36] World Health Organization. ICF, International Classification of Functioning, Disability and Health. Geneva: World Health Organization; 2001

[37] Canadian Interprofessional Health Collaborative. A National Interprofessional Competency Framework. Vancouver, British Columbia: College of Health Disciplines, University of British Columbia; 2010

[38] Nelson A, Iwama M. Cultural influences and occupation-centred practice with children and families. In: Rodger S, ed. Occupation-Centred Practice with Children: A Practical Guide for Occupational Therapists. Oxford: Wiley-Blackwell; 2010:75–93

[39] Christiansen C, Baum C. Enabling Function and Well-Being. 2nd ed. Thorofare, NJ: Slack; 1997

Index

Index